BODY BEAUTIFUL

Oscar Heidenstam

Illustrated by John Babbage

W. FOULSHAM & CO. LTD.

LONDON · NEW YORK · TORONTO · CAPE TOWN · SYDNEY

W. FOULSHAM & COMPANY LIMITED
Yeovil Road, Slough, Berkshire, SL1 4JH

ISBN 0-572-01256-X

Photoset in Great Britain by
C. R. Barber & Partners (Highlands) Ltd., Fort William,
Scotland
and printed by St Edmundsbury Press,
Bury St Edmunds, Suffolk

CONTENTS

FOREWORD

As a physiotherapist, I welcome Oscar Heidenstam's book on all-round exercise for women, and approve the emphasis he has given to weight resisted movements.

In most physical medicine departments of hospitals, muscle re-education by means of weight training exercises has become routine practice, but until recently such treatment was largely confined to male patients. It has been found, however, that properly applied weight training and progressive exercises are equally beneficial to women.

Oscar Heidenstam has dealt with all these points in a thorough and scientific manner. He has had a fine reputation in the physical culture world for many years and has made a specialised study of weight training in all its aspects. His knowledge of anatomy and physiology is sound and his exercise schemes for women have been medically approved. I can guarantee that no woman need have second thoughts about using any of the routines in this book.

On the contrary, many famous women – dancers, actresses and athletes – have found that resistance exercises are the quickest, surest and most accurate way of adding or subtracting centimetres and improving health and figure beauty.

From a therapeutic point of view, I have found that resistance exercises are twice as effective as freestanding exercises, and beneficial results are reached in a much shorter time. Freestanding exercises, however, are useful for promoting tone, suppleness and general fitness, and should be included in every exercise scheme, particularly for older women.

I have practised in industry for many years, and have treated a great many office workers who spend most of their day crouched over desks in stuffy offices. These people suffer postural strains and tension symptoms; resistance exercises are ideal for them.

Books on resistance exercises for men have been around for some time; now, at last, here is an important book for women.

Diana Saunders MCSP *King's College Hospital, London*

INTRODUCTION

Not many years ago it would have been unthinkable for a woman to take up resistance exercises. That kind of thing was reserved for bodybuilding athletes. But times have changed. In recent years men in all walks of life have discovered that progressive resistance, or weight training, exercises can be employed to promote all-round bodily well-being – and not just to build big muscles and great strength. Women, too, have found they can retain health, youth and beauty by exercising with light barbells and dumbells.

What can you, an average woman, gain from these exercises?

1. You can reduce or put on weight where you need it, and so improve your figure. The stimulating exercise will bring radiant health, and health in its turn will bring better looks and lasting youth.

2. If you play games you can take a leaf from the book of many famous sportswomen and employ resistance exercises specifically designed to improve your sport.

3. If you have some postural defect (and so many people have) you can do remedial exercises to remedy it. For many years physiotherapists have been using pulleys and sandbags to give patients exercise. This is weight training in a non-scientific way. But modern progressive resistance techniques are far more accurate and give quicker results.

By the way, please don't be put off by those phrases 'weight lifting' and 'weight training', or by talk of barbells and dumbells. I know it does, unfortunately, conjure up a picture of an old-time strong man with giant muscles, curly moustache, leopard skin and gladiator boots. Progressive resistance exercise (a long-winded way of saying weight training) is smooth and gentle, the weights involved are light and there is no strain.

I want you to try it under my guidance. We will work together, step by step. Soon you will feel fitter than you have ever been in your life. You will really start living.

The physical work involved will be fairly easy, but you will need moral courage, because well-meaning friends, when they hear about what you are doing, will try to put you off. We are all a bit lazy at heart and like to excuse ourselves from exercising – or find excuses to stop other people.

They will say you will develop big muscles. They will say you will strain your heart, or get varicose veins. They will say you'll get fat. If you are an athlete, they will say weight training slows you down. Nonsense!

Today's women athletes, so many of them weight trainers, are mostly slim, glamorous and extremely feminine young ladies. The day of the 'horsey' sportswoman has long gone. Even top athletes, gymnasts and skaters can look attrative and have feminine figures.

Our modern sportswomen train scientifically. They glow with good health and enjoy life to the full. No wonder they are so attractive to look at. And as for weak hearts and varicose veins. Well, as I said, nonsense!

Get this clear. You don't have to be a fanatic. You don't have to deny yourself all the pleasures of life to be fit. But once you are really fit, you will enjoy those pleasures all the more – and without taxing your youth, looks or figure.

Your age does not matter. It is never too late to start. The only important thing is to make sure your exercise programme suits your particular age and level of fitness – in other words, take it gently. I want you to spend forty-five minutes, three times a week, on simple progressive resistance exercises. That is all you need to keep your youth and figure. Surely this is far easier than hours spent in beauty parlours, sauna baths and massage clinics. It is certainly far better than starving yourself on rigid diets which only make you feel hungry and depressed, or doping yourself with slimming pills – that way you ruin your health and lose your youth and looks.

If you are under twenty-one you probably take your vitality and beauty for granted, but in your twenties, the lines and wrinkles start to appear, you become less supple and less able to enjoy life. It's no good hiding the wrinkles with cosmetics and excuse your laziness by saying, 'Well, I'm getting older'. Only two things will help you to retain your looks and figure – regular exercise and sensible diet.

If you are thin, exercise will build you up. If you are fat, exercise will fine you down. You can take centimetres off one place and put them on another. It can all be done with weight training, plus bending and stretching to keep you supple and agile.

I have mentioned that many famous sportswomen use weight training exercises, so do film stars, actresses and models. Entertainer Marti Caine used to enter figure contests and was a member of a women's weight training display team from Sheffield, when in her teens. Actress Linda Evans is one of many film and television stars who have written books of exercise programmes – and she looks better and is fitter and healthier than many teenagers. Olivia Newton John has long been an avid keep-fit fanatic, and so it goes on. You can go into any well known health club and you would be surprised at the famous people who train for their figures. Jane Fonda's book on exercise is a best seller.

Here is an extract from a personal letter written to me by the late Jayne Mansfield, the Hollywood star who was known around the gyms of California long before she became famous on the screen.

There is nothing so important as health. Good health can only be obtained by a combination of beneficial exercises and correct diet. Eternal youth can only be maintained through exercises with weights. I keep my body beautiful by using my husband's barbells, which open the door to health, happiness and success.

There are no short cuts to youth and beauty, but resistance exercise guarantees you the quickest results in the shortest time. That's a certainty.

I hope you are going to try my exercises. I think you owe it to yourself to do so. These are difficult days for women. More and more they are doing jobs once thought open only to men – and yet keeping a home going as well. All this takes its toll of youth and looks. You just must find the time to look after your health.

With good health will come a good figure and the ability to wear the latest fashions without looking like a scarecrow or bursting at the seams.

I don't care how busy you are. The busiest woman in the world can spare forty-five minutes three times a week. And if you are really that busy, I will cut it down to fifteen minutes twice a week.

In return you will get something money cannot buy. You owe it to yourself. If you are married, you owe it to your husband and the future generation.

Chapter 1

HEALTH

Modern life is tough and complex. It makes great demands on our physical and mental stamina. Today, the health service is one of the nation's greatest expenses. Doctors' waiting-rooms are filled with patients waiting for the inevitable prescription for some nervous complaint. So many people have nothing actually organically wrong with them, but they are always tired and listless and full of aches and pains. Thousands of working hours are lost to industry every day because of minor ailments.

What is the matter with us? It is simply that we are not bothering to take normal care of our bodies.

Accidents will always happen, and no matter how careful we are some serious illnesses cannot be avoided. But if we keep fit we will be less accident-prone and infection will find it harder to break through our defences. Let yourself drop below par and you fall an easy victim to disease germs. You catch every cold that is going, and vague headaches, backaches and nervous troubles are always interfering with your everyday life.

You just cannot afford to go on being only half alive. You may have a career before you, or you may have a house to run and children to bring up. Like so many women today you may be coping with both a career and a home.

There is no doubt about it. A woman must be really fit to keep up with the pace of modern life, and only when she is fit will she realise how much it means.

Fitness is not such a difficult goal, if you will take the trouble to learn something about your body and how to keep it in perfect working order with the minimum of effort.

Yet so very many women can't, or won't, bother. They sadly resign themselves to middle-age when hardly out of their twenties. They have two children and let themselves go. They suffer bad teeth, poor complexions, varicose veins, aching feet, postural defects and all sorts of minor ailments. They just don't know how to take care of their bodies.

It's strange, isn't it? Women are traditionally more conscious of their looks and figure than are men, yet men have been much quicker to realise the benefits of regular and progressive exercise to keep the body looking and feeling on the top line.

I must repeat this over and over again, because it is so very important. Cosmetics and pills cannot restore your looks, retard premature old age, bring back supple curves and that youthful sparkle in your eyes. Only good health can do that, and good health can only be achieved through fitness.

Let me prove my point with a few examples. Have you ever considered the careers of some of the world's great dancers? Many of them are still at the height of their physical powers though well past fifty. They have beautiful figures, sparkling eyes, lovely complexions – their grace and deportment delight millions. Why do they keep so young? Because all their lives they have kept in perfect condition with exercise. The answer is as easy as that.

We will not delve into exact ages, but the great Anna Pavlova was at the height of her career when nearly sixty. Alicia Markova was a star for thirty years, and still teaches. Margot Fonteyn was dancing in star roles until she was sixty.

Yes, I can hear you say it now. These great ballerinas devote their lives to their art – they spend hours every day keeping fit. So they do. But I have no intention of training you to be a great ballerina. I just want you to be fit and healthy to enjoy life to the full, and I can achieve that result if you will give me forty-five minutes three times a week to do simple exercises.

Your body is a machine. All machines need regular attention. Yet a woman will abuse her body and ignore all the elementary rules of maintenance. Then she wonders why her looks suffer. She wonders why she is beginning to look older than her years.

What are the main causes of premature ageing? Here they are.

1. Faulty diet. There's no need to fuss about diet. But try and cut down those odd cups of tea with sugar. Don't make do with coffee and a cigarette when you should be eating a square meal. And if you live in a bed-sitter you are probably opening too many tins and taking meals consisting largely of starches and carbohydrates.

2. Lack of exercise. You walk to the bus daily, amble in the park occasionally when it's fine, swim when on holiday. It's not enough. Household chores are not sufficient either. You need carefully designed exercise.

3. Poor personal hygiene. Of course you should take plenty of

baths and clean your teeth at least twice a day. And no matter how late to bed you are after a special evening, always remove all make-up and wash your face and neck before going to bed.

4. Lack of sleep. Late nights once in a while are fine, but don't make a habit of it. Your body needs sound sleep to restore itself. Sound sleep, without the aids of sedatives, only comes with good health.

5. Faulty posture. Many jobs create postural defects, and nothing shows your age more than the way you stand and walk. Exercises can do a lot for posture. Don't wear tight shoes. And try not to wear shoes with too high a heel. Aching feet show in your face, remember.

6. Mental outlook. A woman is as old as she feels – never forget that. If you are fit and in good health you will feel young and you will look young.

7. Bad habits. It is easier to start smoking and drinking than to stop. If you haven't yet started, for goodness sake don't. If you have, start by cutting down and do your best to cut it out.

Chapter 2

VITAL STATISTICS

You have a great deal of control over your weight and body measurements, but you are limited by your particular 'physical type'. I want to tell you a little about this, partly because it will help you in your quest for health and beauty, and also because it will prevent you from trying to achieve the impossible.

Your physical type depends largely on your bone structure, and there are three main types. These are known as ectomorph, mesomorph and endomorph, and the meanings are quite simple. The ectomorph is light-boned, the mesomorph is medium-boned and of athletic build, the endomorph is big-boned and naturally stout.

If we go back to Greek mythology we can find excellent examples of these three types. Aphrodite, the goddess of love, was an ectomorph, small and light-boned. Diana, the huntress, was the slender and athletic mesomorph. While the Venus de Milo, with her large hips and heavy build, was the typical endomorph.

Many women, of course, are a mixture of more than one type. Their upper bodies may be small and light-boned yet they may have thick legs and hips. But most women (and men, too, for that matter) come within the three main types.

Your type depends on ancestry, environment and many other vital factors. You are unlikely to change it, so you should be aware of your physical type and of the restrictions it places on your 'ideal' figure. If you are big-boned, you will never be a sylph, even if you starve yourself and ruin your health. For you, it's getting the centimetres and curves in the right places that's going to count.

Now let's take a closer look at the three main types and see how they measure up both physically and emotionally; because there is something in the old wives' tale; your physical build does to some extent condition your temperament and outlook on life and modern athletics coaches, for instance, make important use of this in training. Remember, however, that these are generalisations and should be viewed with that in mind.

Generally speaking, I have found that the light-boned girl has a small bust, and her hip measurement is slightly larger than her bust. Although she may be slim and light-boned, the structure of her pelvis is such that her hips are fairly wide compared with her other measurements.

The naturally thin, light-boned girl is more likely to be highly strung. She burns up a great deal of nervous energy and finds it hard to gain weight. She eats all she likes and still keeps the same weight because she is using energy quicker than she can replace it.

The medium-boned girl is physically an athletic type, even though she may not play games or have any interest in sport. She has long legs, a trim waist and hip measurements smaller than her bust. She has little or no weight troubles. Most top-line sportswomen, figure contest winners and models come into this category.

This girl usually has a placid nature and is not a worrier.

The heavy-boned girl is often not really large in the bust, but her bone structure gives her this appearance. Her waist tends to be thick and she has heavy hips and thighs. She certainly gains weight easily.

This girl tends to be sluggish and dislikes moving about more than is absolutely necessary.

By now, I am sure you will want to know your own type and find out whether you are an ectomorph, a mesomorph or an endomorph. The medical people do a lot of complicated measuring with calipers, but a good guide is to examine the formation of your ribs where they separate. A very narrow angle between the two sets of ribs indicates the small-boned type. A rather wider angle would make you medium-boned. And a very wide angle, forming almost a semi-circle in some people, is the mark of the heavy-boned type. Wrist and ankle measurements are also a good guide, as they are not likely to increase in size once adult (except by injury or disease, of course).

Now look at the guide on page 14. It may differ slightly from other guides because it is only a guide. It has been compiled from my own extensive knowledge of the measurements of beauty contest winners over the last few years and should give you some help in assessing your figure.

You will see that there is very little variation in measurements for women of different heights but of similar bone structure. But you will also see that body weight varies considerably according to bone structure. In fact, two women of the same height, both having ideal proportions for their physical type, can vary in weight by as much as 9 kg (20 lb). That is what I meant when I said that a knowledge of physical types would prevent your trying to achieve the impossible.

Your weight for your height will vary considerably according to your type. But it's how you look that counts. Progressive resistance exercise and a carefully planned diet will give you the best measurements and weight for your height and type, and then you will look your best.

You will notice that my chart of 'ideal' measurements only covers the age group from twenty to thirty-five years old, but the modern woman remains thirty-five in spirit and looks for at least ten years after she has passed that birthday. Even though she bears and raises a family, her figure need only show a slight fullness with the passing of time.

I mentioned earlier that some women are a mixture of types. There is the small-boned woman with the exceptionally large bust, or the large-boned woman with thin lower legs and ankles. These cases can be difficult. But the specialised exercises I am going to describe can be used to improve just the bad points in any individual figure, and it is surprising just how big an improvement can be made.

I cannot close this chapter without a mention of that strange phenomenon of the mid-twentieth century, the 'cult of the bosom'. This subject still fills thousands of pages of photographs and comments in magazines, from the seaside to streakers. It is big news in the media; page 3 in a national newspaper is one of its best selling items! Perhaps with more women prepared to go topless, even in public places, we might in time lose interest.

What the press agents conveniently forget (or, more likely, don't know) is that the young ladies in question are always heavy-boned and have wide shoulders. Their upper bodies are endomorphic and so their bust measurements may be little more than above average for that physical type.

However, whatever nature provided you with – whether large or small – a firm and attractive bust is something most women desire. Exercise is the finest way to help you, this is guaranteed. Exercise may not increase the size of your bust, but it will increase the size of your rib cage, and therefore make your bust look much better shaped, and firmer.

A GUIDE TO MEASUREMENTS

These figures refer to women between twenty and thirty-five years of age. They are not meant to be ideal, but just a guide with which to make some comparison. Many experts have different ideas of 'ideal' measurements, and even of correct weight.

HEIGHT	1 m 52 cm– 1 m 55 cm (5 ft–5 ft 1 in)	1 m 57 cm– 1 m 60 cm (5 ft 2 in–5 ft 3 in)	1 m 63 cm– 1 m 65 cm (5 ft 4 in–5 ft 5 in)	1 m 68 cm– 1 m 70 cm (5 ft 6 in–5 ft 7 in)	1 m 73 cm– 1 m 75 cm (5 ft 8 in–5 ft 9 in)
SMALL BONED (ECTOMORPH)					
Bust	84 cm (33 in)	85 cm (33½ in)	86 cm (34 in)	89 cm (35 in)	90 cm (35½ in)
Waist	56 cm (22 in)	57 cm (22½ in)	58 cm (23 in)	60 cm (23½ in)	60 cm (23½ in)
Hips	85 cm (33½ in)	86 cm (34 in)	88 cm (34½ in)	90 cm (35½ in)	91 cm (36 in)
MEDIUM BONED (MESOMORPH)					
Bust	88 cm (34½ in)	89 cm (35 in)	91 cm (36 in)	93 cm (36½ in)	94 cm (37 in)
Waist	56 cm (22 in)	57 cm (22½ in)	58 cm (23 in)	60 cm (23½ in)	61 cm (24 in)
Hips	86 cm (34 in)	88 cm (34½ in)	89 cm (35 in)	91 cm (36 in)	91 cm (36 in)
LARGE BONED (ENDOMORPH)					
Bust	89 cm (35 in)	90 cm (35½ in)	93 cm (36½ in)	95 cm (37½ in)	98 cm (38½ in)
Waist	58 cm (23 in)	60 cm (23½ in)	61 cm (24 in)	62 cm (24½ in)	64 cm (25 in)
Hips	89 cm (35 in)	90 cm (35½ in)	91 cm (36 in)	93 cm (36½ in)	97 cm (38 in)

Chapter 3

MUSCLES AND EXERCISE

When I was a child, a nursery rhyme said that little boys were made of slugs and snails and puppy dogs' tails, and little girls were made of sugar and spice and all things nice.

It is a picturesque thought. Who knows, it may have encouraged generations of women in the belief that their physical structure is vastly different from that of the male of the species. This in turn may have led them to think that while exercise is permissible for a man, it is unladylike, unnecessary and dangerous for a woman.

In actual fact the physical differences between men and women are very few. The skeletal and muscular systems are identical; as are the circulatory, respiratory and nervous systems.

A woman's skeletal and general structure, of course, is usually smaller than a man's; her pelvis is wider and her knees less knobbly. She has a longer body and shorter legs and is heavier round the hips, tops of the thighs and the bust. Her rib formation gives her less lung capacity than a man. There are certainly marked differences in the glandular system and from these differences she derives her female emotions and psychology.

Some women are rather scared of the word 'muscles'. Perhaps they feel it is not a very feminine word. But whether they like it or not, women do possess muscles – and those muscles occupy 36 per cent of their total physical make-up. A man has rather more muscle and proportionately less fatty tissue.

Professor R. D. Lockhart, MD, ChM, a famous author on the subject, in his book *Living Anatomy*, gave these comparative figures:

Fatty tissue in women 28 per cent; in men 18 per cent.

Muscles in women 36 per cent; in men 42 per cent.

Whether muscles belong to a male or a female, they have one quality in common. If they are not used, they turn to fatty tissue or they atrophy, so they must be exercised.

A woman can exercise her muscles quite considerably and still remain entirely feminine. She has a naturally thicker layer of fatty tissue just below the skin surface, so instead of her physique becoming hard and muscular, it takes on a firm and healthy quality and loses all those unsightly wrinkles and fat on legs, waist, hips and bust.

The exercises I am going to give you in this book have all been designed to work your muscles through their full range of movement. If a muscle is continually worked through a limited range it becomes shortened. This impairs the movement of the joint to which it is attached. And that is what some people still call the old chestnut 'muscle bound'. This unfortunate term has nothing to do with fully trained muscles. You can be muscle bound, without ever having done an exercise in your life.

People in factories or doing certain types of manual work, office workers sitting at desks for long hours, can all become muscle bound if they take no exercise to compensate for time spent standing or sitting in fixed positions.

Office workers, in particular, often develop round shoulders, shortened chest and shoulder muscles while their abdominal muscles are weakened. The weaker the muscles, and the more fat they put on, the more open they are to defects of this sort.

The constant wearing of high heels causes postural defects and shortened muscles because the body is thrown out of normal balance and the pelvis is tilted. This does not mean that a woman should not wear fashionable shoes, but it does mean that she must keep herself in good trim to minimise ill effects.

In this chapter I have concentrated on muscles and how they are affected by exercise, but correctly prescribed exercise has a beneficial effect on the entire body.

The heart is strengthened by regular exercise (and the heart is a muscle, remember). The respiratory system is given increased efficiency, more oxygen is fed to the blood and this in turn brings improved circulation. Blood vessels in their thousands reach out to all parts of the muscular system. Because exercise boosts the circulation it ensures that the muscles are fed and nourished by an adequate blood supply.

Deep within us all there is an urge to exercise. It is there in the healthy child 'on the go' from morning till night. It is there in the young man or woman's urge to excel at athletics and in the old person's desire to stimulate the circulation by taking a mild stroll.

A very famous physical culturist, Eugene Sandow, once said that, 'life is movement'. If we allow ourselves to become sluggish and lazy we deteriorate mentally as well as physically.

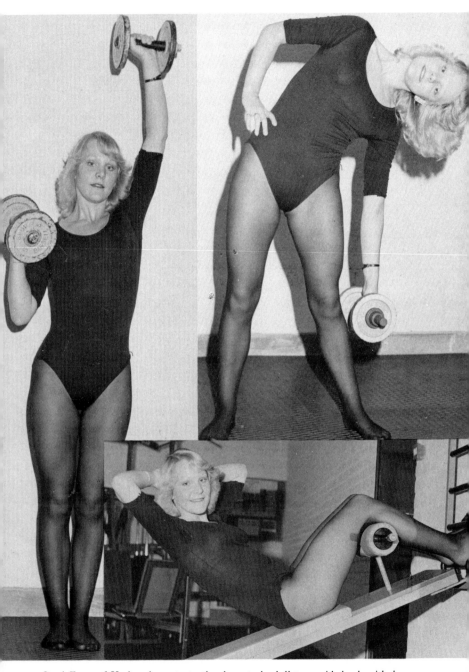

Carol Evans of Harlow demonstrates the alternate dumbell press, side bends with dumbells, and sit ups. Carol has herself won many figure contests. She enjoys training, and the feeling of fitness it gives her.

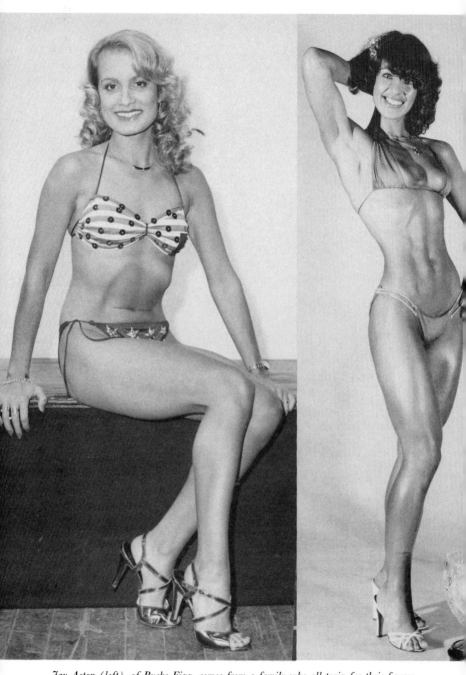

Jay Aston (left), of Bucks Fizz, comes from a family who all train for their figures. Her grandfather was once Britain's Strongest Man. She has entered many figure contests.

Here is proof that childbirth need not mean goodbye to your figure – Mary Scott (right) has three children. Besides being a housewife, she has a part-time job as well as doing some modelling.

Chapter 4

SANE EATING FOR GOOD HEALTH

Possibly more nonsense has been written on the subject of diet than practically any other aspect of human health. It is not surprising that the average woman, bewildered by conflicting advice in every magazine she picks up, begins to wonder if the so-called experts really know anything at all. More books and magazine articles have been written on diet than almost any other subject. Read them by all means, but try and draw your own conclusions when you have tried exercise to go with your diet.

Most of us eat too much. That is a fairly safe statement to make on a subject which bristles with contradictions. The trouble is that we don't eat the right foods. Amazing though it may sound, it is quite possible for a fat person to be suffering from malnutrition.

Women are, unfortunately, particularly prone to try the new fad of the moment. Some of these diets are cranky but harmless. Others, though, are positively dangerous if followed for any length of time. And a woman, determined to lose pounds quickly, will gaily reduce herself to near starvation, ruin her health, shred her nerves and, in the process, lose whatever good looks she may have possessed.

Let me give you a warning right away. Don't go on any rigid diet unless your doctor prescribes it. Sensible eating, combined with regular exercise, is all the average woman needs for health and good looks.

You require different foods to supply the body's varying needs. You must have food to supply fuel for energy and warmth, to build up new tissue and repair old tissue, and to regulate the substances which control the complex machinery of the body.

Certain foods are essential. You need them whether you want to lose or gain weight, or remain the same. Without them you will not be healthy. The essential items of our diet are proteins, carbohydrates, fats, vitamins, minerals and water. Let us take a closer look at each in turn.

PROTEINS

The word 'protein' means 'first' and is an indication of the importance of the foods within this group. Proteins help to replace and repair the muscular tissue broken down by normal bodily functions. They are the main sources of energy and certain essential minerals.

The best protein foods are milk, eggs, fish, poultry, cheese (especially cottage cheese) and lean meat. To a lesser degree protein is also contained in vegetables – particularly, beans, peas, carrots, spinach and cabbage. Soya beans and soya flour, are the main constituents of most proprietary protein foods.

With the exception of milk and some cheeses, none of these foods is particularly high in calories. Make sure that your daily diet contains an adequate amount of at least two or three of these items. They are essential to health.

Milk is considered to be the most nearly perfect food. It provides babies with all their nourishment but it is not in itself an adequate diet for an adult. Even so, 600 ml (1 pt) of milk can provide a quarter of your daily protein requirement. The equivalent would be one good portion of fish or lean meat or two eggs.

CARBOHYDRATES

These supply the body's fuel. They are found mainly in sugars and starches.

Most people tend to take too much carbohydrate in the form of bread, cake, pastry and potatoes. But beware of any diet which is completely deficient in carbohydrate; it will make you listless and lifeless. Wholemeal bread is an excellent source.

The sugars in your diet will come from honey, syrup, fruit and glucose. Natural sugars and molasses are better for you than refined products which are little more than 'empty calories'. Glucose is easily taken into the blood stream.

FATS

They are similar in structure to the carbohydrates. Animal sources are butter, meat, bacon and milk. Certain fish – herring and sardine, for instance – are rich in fat. Margarine, peanut butter and olive oil are good vegetable sources. There are also small quantities in cheese and eggs.

VITAMINS

The term is derived from the word 'life'. There is still a lot to be learned about vitamins and their effect on the human body. We do know that they are essential to health, and we know the foods in which they are found.

Only very small quantities of vitamins are needed and a well-balanced diet covering the three essentials already mentioned should also include them. Some people suffer from vitamin deficiency, and vitamin tablets can put this right. But if you lack vitamins it is a sure warning that something is wrong with your daily diet.

Vitamin A is necessary for general health and growth. Lack of it can lead to rough skin and respiratory troubles. The main sources are liver, leafy vegetables, yellow vegetables, cheese, egg yolk and fruit.

Vitamin B is a complex substance sub-divided into groups but, for the purpose of healthy eating, we can look at it as one. Lack of vitamin B leads to fatigue, diseases of the nervous system, mental and digestive troubles and constipation. It is found in lean meat, cereals, beans, cheese and some vegetables. Yeast is a good source and is often prescribed by doctors in tablet form for patients displaying symptoms of vitamin B deficiency.

Vitamin C is necessary to guard against anaemia, depression, rough skin, poor gums and the common cold. Vitamin C is generally known as ascorbic acid. The main sources are citrus fruits, tomatoes and many other pulpy fruits.

Vitamin D is sometimes called the 'sunshine vitamin' because it is formed by the action of ultra-violet light on our skins. Lack of it leads to poor teeth and bone structure and makes us less resistant to colds and infection. It is found in eggs, milk, cream and fish oil. Halibut oil and cod liver oil are well known sources.

Vitamin E is commonly known as the 'vitality and fertility vitamin', which adequately describes its qualities. It can be used in cooking with wheat germ oil, or found in whole grain cereals, lettuce, broccoli and Brussels sprouts.

MINERALS

Iron and calcium are essential to the making of blood and bone. They are found in milk, dairy produce, brown bread, vegetables and fruit. Sulphur and phosphorus are found in many foods, including common salt.

There are many other minerals which the body requires to function efficiently, but these are needed in such minute amounts that they should be adequate in a healthy, balanced diet.

WATER

About two-thirds of your total body weight is fluid. Sufficient water is essential for the proper functioning of the kidneys and to ensure regular elimination.

Do remember that water is not only for washing. It is not very interesting stuff but you should drink at least 1.5 litres (3 pt) a day. It won't make you fat. And a glass of warm water and lemon first thing every day is better than any laxative.

LOSING WEIGHT

I said at the start of this chapter that you should not go on a rigid diet unless told to by a doctor, and I mean that. How, then, you may ask, can you adjust your diet to lose weight?

There is no mystery about it at all. Cut down your food intake generally, but make sure that you are getting enough protein, vitamins and so on to keep you healthy. In other words, follow a good, balanced diet but eat slightly less than you would normally.

Cut down on starches and carbohydrates – less bread, less potatoes, less sugar. Cut down on fats – poached egg for breakfast instead of fried, cottage cheese instead of Cheddar. Cut down on those extra cups of tea. Instead, eat more fresh food, especially fruit and vegetables.

Note that I say 'cut down', not cut out altogether. There is no need to be a martyr. In fact, a diet which makes you feel listless and constantly hungry is guaranteed to fail, since you will be always thinking about food and are much more likely to sneak the odd biscuit or abandon the diet altogether. Regulate your diet on these simple lines, do some of the exercises I am going to tell you about and you will reduce gradually and safely.

Your body is a complex piece of machinery. Rob it of fuel and it will not function correctly. So I repeat, don't try to starve yourself.

I cannot tell you exactly what to eat and when to eat it; individuals vary so considerably. One woman may thrive on two large meals a day. Another woman may need frequent small snacks. But it is a good idea to try to eat at the same times every day. I know this can be difficult, but the stomach is very much a creature of habit. If you possibly can, I advise you to indulge your stomach on this point.

Avoid 'nibbling' between meals. Skipping a wholesome breakfast then having two biscuits with your coffee is no good for anyone. Also try to avoid heavy meals late in the evening, as your body does not have time to use up the calories.

Take some care in the preparation of food. Don't overcook it and destroy its natural goodness. Avoid frying – grill, steam, poach or bake instead. Don't eat warmed-up leftovers – fresh, well cooked food has far more nutritional value.

Give yourself time to eat a meal. Food should be eaten slowly and well masticated. Rushed meals are one of the greatest single causes of digestive troubles and constipation.

There is no such thing as a miracle-working diet that will solve your health and weight problems in a couple of weeks. If you have been following a bad diet for years, you cannot expect your body to adjust overnight, so the sooner you start, the better – and don't give up. If your diet is unbalanced, too high in fats, refined carbo-hydrates and 'junk' foods, then the only answer is to change it.

Eat according to the suggestions I have made, watch those fats and carbohydrates, do the exercises which are going to come, and health and figure beauty will be yours.

It will take a little time before you begin to see results. But there will certainly be results. And as the months go by, and you check your progress in the mirror and on the bathroom scales – as well as simply by the way you feel – I think you will come to agree that sensible eating and a little scientific exercise are not such bad things after all.

DIET SUMMARY

To set a daily diet sheet is complex, as a great deal depends on the foods in season, what you can afford, your personal needs, and what you enjoy.

Unless you are taking exercise, cut down on food generally. Those who are overweight or underweight may find the following lists of what they can eat helpful.

FOR REDUCING

Lean meat, poultry, fish (not fried or oily fish), eggs (not more than two a day), cheese (limited).

Oranges, grapefruit, apples, plums, rhubarb, berries – better than tinned or stewed fruit.

Salads, cabbage, spinach, tomatoes (as much as you like).

Beans, peas, carrots (not so much as the other vegetables).

Wholemeal bread (preferably toasted), about 4 – 5 slices a day.

Cereals, Ryvita and wheat biscuits.

Butter (limited), sugar (unrefined, limited), low fat, high polyunsaturated margarine (preferable to butter or ordinary margarine).

Honey and natural sugars (better than jams, etc.).

Limit the following:
Fried foods, i.e. chips, fried eggs, bacon, sausages, etc.

Sweets, i.e. pastries, cakes, chocolates.

Starches, i.e. potatoes, pastry, spaghetti, etc.

Beverages, i.e. tea, milky coffee, beer, spirits.

Sauces and spices, i.e. mayonnaise, white sauce, olive oil, etc.

Milk, restrict to 300 ml ($\frac{1}{2}$ pt) daily for all uses.

Butter or margarine 50 g (2 oz) daily.

A typical diet could be:
Glass of orange or lemon juice – hot or cold according to season – unsweetened.

Breakfast: Grapefruit, boiled egg, two pieces of wholemeal toast, thin spread of butter, marmalade, one cup of tea or coffee – little milk and one teaspoonful of brown sugar.

Mid-morning: Fresh fruit drink.

Lunch: Meat or fish (not fried), or hard boiled egg, salad, plenty of cabbage or spinach, two small potatoes (boiled or creamed); apple, or orange, or both, or freshly stewed fruit not too sweet.

Tea: One cup of tea and biscuits, or one slice of plain cake.

Supper or high tea: Poached egg, or lean meat, or cold meat, salad or green vegetables, no potatoes; milk pudding or fruit; or yoghurt – this can be taken at breakfast if preferred.

FOR GAINING

Eat almost anything, but still limit fried foods, pastries, rich cakes, etc.

Include extra milk – at least 600 ml (1 pt) a day – chocolate, ice-cream, bananas, extra cheese and eggs, plenty of butter, honey, treacle, nuts, raisins. Olive oil, halibut oil, or cod liver oil and malt can also be taken.

HEALTH FOODS

So-called 'health foods' are a multi-million pound business, and every week some new miracle 'pill' appears. Nearly every reputable chemist has a 'health food' counter, and specialist shops flourish. They sell two main kinds of product: healthy foods, such as wholemeal bread and flours, natural yoghurt, nuts, fruits, and so on; and food supplements, such as vitamin pills, which are designed to supplement your normal diet with essential vitamins and minerals which you may be lacking.

Everyone should eat more healthy foods, rather than the fatty, over-sweet 'junk' foods which comprise such a large proportion of our diet, but most of these are readily available in supermarkets and ordinary shops and probably cost less there. Among the healthiest foods are fresh fruit and vegetables, which really makes the term 'health food' a misnomer.

The majority of normal, healthy people who follow a good balanced diet should obtain all the necessary nutrients from their food without the need for supplements, although they do have an important place in any health plan, and are invaluable for sportspeople and those involved in heavy physical work, and are ideal as an extra 'tonic' to be used after illness, for example.

But what do you take? The variety of food supplements is inexhaustible, as are the makers, and the advertised advantages of some products are unproven. It is therefore wise to use only supplements of proven value, and a good coach should be able to define your specific needs. A good protein drink, for example, made with milk, is ideal if you are run down, but remember that too much milk is fattening, so cut the milk if you are trying to lose weight. If you cannot afford to buy best steaks, then such items as concentrated liver tablets are excellent. Wheatgerm capsules are ideal for extra vitamin E, and so on.

Generally speaking, doctors are reticent about the advantages and disadvantages of advertised health foods, probably because there are so many, and they feel that some are phoney. Yet everyone realises the importance of obtaining essential vitamins – doctors often prescribe extra vitamin B, for example, for convalescence. The important thing is to be sceptical of the so-called 'miracle workers', but be aware of the advantages and the place of recognised food supplements in your diet.

In general, most common food supplements are harmless, but you should always follow recommended doses. Most people will not feel the need to use them, but for athletes, in special circumstances, and when fresh vegetables and good foods are expensive or hard to obtain, dietary supplements can play an important role in keeping you healthy.

Chapter 5

INTRODUCTION TO YOUR EXERCISE PLAN

On previous pages I have talked a lot about the importance of exercise. In this chapter I shall give you a few general do's and don't's and then we will be ready to get down to work.

How often should you exercise? For best results I suggest you make a real effort to exercise not less than three times a week. That may require a little rearrangement of your activities but I think you will find it well worth the trouble.

If you just cannot manage three times a week, you will have to make do with less, but the exercise must be regular. It is no use at all being terribly keen and exercising five times in one week and then doing nothing at all the following two weeks. The essentials for physical improvement are: continuity, progression and correct performance of every exercise attempted.

At what time of the day should you exercise? Whatever time you choose try to make it the same time every exercise day. Your stomach prefers its food at regular times, and your body feels the same way about exercise.

Whatever the old physical jerks school of instructors may say, first thing in the morning is not a good time. For most people the best time is somewhere between your evening meal and going to bed, or before your evening meal, if you prefer it that way.

Some women, I well realise, will have to exercise in the mornings. They may work in the evenings, or they may be housewives who find they have most time to spare after their husbands have gone off to work and the children have been taken to school. But, I repeat, none of this leaping out of bed first thing in the morning and starting to exercise. Your body won't appreciate it and you will derive very little benefit.

Where should you exercise? The best place is a warm but well-ventilated room. Exercise in the freezing cold does nobody any good, whatever they may have told your husband to the contrary in the army. You want plenty of fresh air without draughts.

If the weather is warm and sunny, and you have a secluded

garden, by all means exercise in the open air. But don't try to be a tough guy in the cold weather.

What clothes should you wear? You will need some form of support, particularly if you are on the stout side, but leave off tight garments and belts and anything which will hinder free movement. There are many attractive leotards available. Most are of a naturally stretchy material and are ideal for your exercises as they are comfortable and give good support. Some are full length to cover the legs, or you can buy footless tights, and this too is good, especially in winter and to avoid leg strains. Heavily built women are better with a full length leotard.

Shorts and a jersey of some kind or a T-shirt are also much used, but shorts can be restricting round the waist, and T-shirts may need extra support if you are heavily built.

You must feel free and comfortable when you exercise, this is important. A gym is not a fashion salon, it is a workroom to improve your figure and looks.

Bare feet to train in are fine, but some gymnasia prefer that you wear some footwear. Light pull-on gym slippers or dancing slippers are not too expensive. Whatever you wear must be light, flexible and flat-heeled.

For a start you will probably be content with a few simple exercises to tone-up the system and keep you in good trim. But I feel that once you have experienced the benefit to be obtained from this work you will want to progress to more advanced weight training exercises.

But whatever your eventual schedule of work, always start every session with a few light limbering-up exercises. This applies, as a matter of fact, to every form of athletic activity. The world champion runner doesn't start his day's training with a four-minute mile. He takes it easy and does some gentle exercise to loosen up. You must apply the same principle to your own exercise routines.

One last point before we really start on the exercises. Only very light exercise should be taken during the monthly period, and, in general, weight training should be avoided at this time.

Chapter 6

EXERCISES WITHOUT APPARATUS

Freestanding exercises, or callisthenics as they are technically termed, are done without any apparatus. Their primary object is a smooth, rhythmical form of movement for all parts of the body, to keep you toned up and supple, and to improve your posture, co-ordination and general stamina.

AEROBICS

This includes the 'aerobics' which is done in health clubs, leisure centres and even dance studios. They are a form of exercises done to disco or other music, and combine free exercises with dance sequences. This form of exercise has been criticised by medical and physical training experts, but anything new often comes in for criticism and suspicion. However, the main complaint is that they are often too strenuous for a complete beginner, and the classes are large, with not enough staff to divide up the trainers into small classes of various standards. Those taking part can be young or old, thin or fat, fairly fit or people who have done no exercise for years. In too many cases you are thrown in at the deep end, and left to fend for yourself at the back of the class. I am sure you have seen it. The good and experienced ones in the front are often not putting in nearly as much effort as they are capable of. The new ones are struggling to keep up and not be shown up, and many are overdoing it.

If you join an aerobics class and have taken no strenuous exercise before, I advise you to do a few weeks of the simple exercises recommended here, and then join the class when you feel fitter.

JOGGING

Jogging is also excellent to get you generally fit, but that too needs caution and even a doctor's recommendation. How far do you go at first? No two people are alike. Also, feet and legs that have only been used to walk to the bus, round the shops or into the car, are often in a very poor state to be bashed on hard roads and pavements. Therefore, if you do take up jogging, take it very slowly and do not do too much. Start by taking a regular walk, then alternate short bursts of slow jogging with walking, gradually increasing the gentle jogging as you feel fitter. If you can jog on a grassy surface, so much the better, and always wear proper jogging shoes. Other clothes are not important as long as your muscles are kept warm and your movements are not restricted, but it is worth paying a little more for a good pair or shoes to protect your feet.

CALLISTHENICS

This form of exercise is ideal for a general fifteen-minute toning up, but progression is limited. Eventually you either have to find harder exercises, or increase the number of repetitions performed.

If you want to increase your strength, or reduce or add weight, you will need something more than freestanding exercises for quick results. With weight training, when you become proficient, you merely increase the resistance by adding weight, thus making the exercises harder.

A good freestanding plan should include exercises for all parts of the body in the following sequence:
1. General light skipping, or running, or small jumps on the spot, to get the circulation working well.
2. Exercises for arms and shoulders, neck, bust and posture.
3. Trunk or body exercises to include back and lateral exercises for strengthening the back and toning the waist.
4. Leg and hip work for co-ordination, balance and trimming thighs and hips.
5. Abdominal exercises to strengthen the mid-section and reduce the tummy, waist and hips.
6. A final breathing exercise for relaxation and to return the system to normal.

There are hundreds of freestanding exercises. Progression is made either by increasing the number of repetitions you perform or by increasing the difficulty of the exercises.

Take, for example, a tummy exercise such as Exercise 15, in

which you lie on your back with your hands at your sides and raise your knees, alternately, to your chest. Progression is made by raising both knees to your chest, as in Exercise 16, or by raising your legs straight, Exercise 17.

I have chosen twenty exercises, which represent every group already mentioned, to make up a ten to fifteen-minute workout, and to allow for progression. You will see that there is a certain amount of overlap in the groups, where tummy exercises also affect the hips and thighs.

I will describe each exercise and you can make up a typical routine by taking one or two exercises from each group.

You can, if you wish, merely pick out individual exercises for parts where you feel exercise is needed most, but it is much better, whatever your personal needs, to have an overall workout for the whole of the body. Everyone finds that they have a strong point, so look for your weaknesses and work that little extra hard on them, but never neglect any part of the body, even when you feel you are already presentable.

Some of these exercises should also be incorporated into your weight training workouts at a later stage.

EXERCISE 1　Practice walking with a book on the head. This is a very old and rather hackneyed exercise, but it will teach you to walk correctly with head erect and shoulders square.

Do it in bare feet or flat-heeled slippers so that you will correct the faults in your posture.

Practise this for a minute or so, concentrating on correct walking with toes pointing straight to the front. Put the foot on the floor in this order: heel, outer arch of foot, toes.

EXERCISES FOR SHOULDERS, ARMS AND POSTURE

EXERCISE 2　Stand astride, arms sideways, fingers pointed straight. Describe small circles backwards, keeping the arms straight. Feel the shoulder blades meeting. Do not stick the tummy out by leaning backwards. Breathe normally. Try twenty small circles, have a breather, and do twenty more.

Progression can be made by increasing the size of the circles until you are circling the arms forwards, upwards and backwards, brushing the ears with the inside of the arms. Always ensure upright posture and no movement of the body.

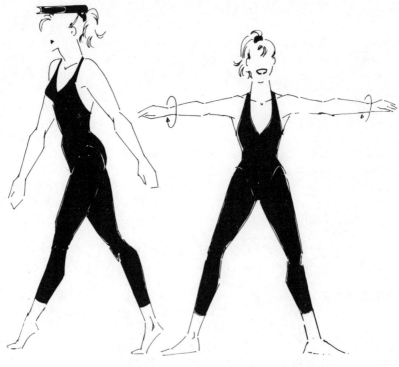

Exercise 1   *Exercise 2*

EXERCISE 3   Stand feet together, arms at sides. Swing the arms sideways and upwards, keeping the fingers pointed. At the same time raise the heels and make yourself as tall as you can. Keep the head well up. Feel the strain on your waist.

Repeat ten times. Rest and repeat again. Breathe in as you lift up, out as you lower the arms.

EXERCISE 4   Stand feet together, arms forward, fingers pointed. Swing the arms forwards and backwards, lowering them slightly below shoulder level as they sweep backwards. Keep the elbows straight and ensure that the movement is confined to the arms and shoulders.

Breathe in as the arms swing sideways and backwards, out as

they return to the starting position. Try ten repetitions, rest, and repeat again.

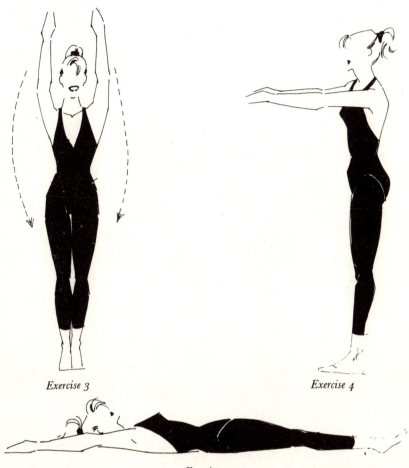

Exercise 3

Exercise 4

Exercise 5

EXERCISE 5 Lie on the back, feet together, toes pointed. Take a heavy book or similar object and place in the palms of the hands. Commence with the arms holding the object above the head, lower it behind the head, keeping the arms straight.

Breathe in as the book is lowered to arms' length behind the head, out as you return to starting position, arms above the head. Repeat ten times, rest, and repeat again. This is a fine shoulder-strengthening exercise.

EXERCISES FOR THE BODY: BACK, WAIST AND HIPS

EXERCISE 6   Stand feet astride. Keeping the knees straight, bend forward to touch alternate toes with opposite arm. Swing the other arm vigorously backwards and upwards. Turn head towards each side. Remain in the forward bend position.

Breathe freely and continue exercise rapidly for a count of thirty. Upward stretch and repeat.

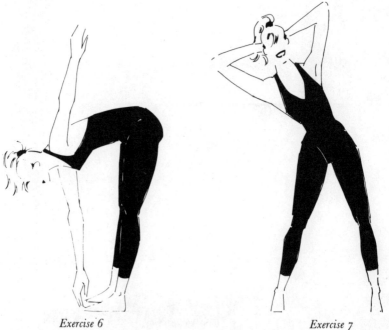

Exercise 6   *Exercise 7*

EXERCISE 7   Stand feet astride, arms in the 'neck rest' position (see illustration), keeping elbows well back. Bend the body from side to side, letting head move freely. Breathe normally. Repeat to count of twenty. Rest and repeat again.

If at first this exercise is a little advanced, commence with feet astride and hands on hips. Progress to above. Further progression can be made by holding the arms straight above the head. Upright carriage should be maintained at all times, and there must be no forward movement of the body.

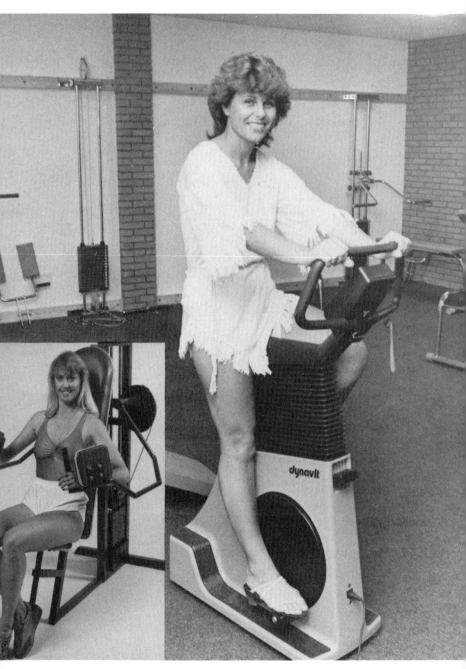

Specialist modern equipment such as the bust exerciser (inset) can be found in many health clubs. Exercise bicycles of all kinds are fairly common and are especially good for the legs.

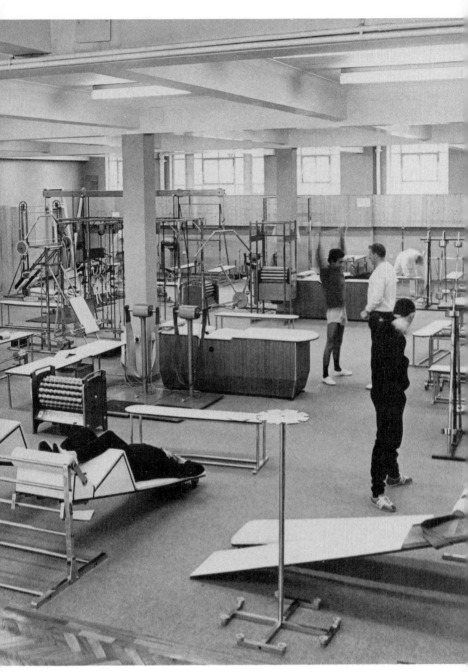

Modern gyms and health clubs are well-equipped to help make training varied and interesting. This is London's Westside Health Club, one of the best known and longest established health clubs.

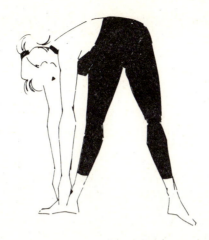

Exercise 8

EXERCISE 8   Stand feet astride. Trunk forward bend and reach down to touch one instep with both hands. Going through the upright position each time, swing over to the opposite side.

Try twelve repetitions in a complete circular movement. Rest and repeat. Breathe normally. Progression can be made by commencing the exercise with arms above the head and returning to starting position.

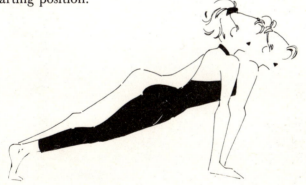

Exercise 9

EXERCISE 9   Support your weight on your two arms, legs straight, body in a straight line from head to toe. Without bending the arms, lower the legs and hips till they touch the floor, lifting the head up high.

Breathe in as you lower the body, out as you return to the starting position. Repeat ten times, rest, and repeat. This exercise is also, of course, a good shoulder and arm strengthener.

EXERCISES FOR HIPS, THIGHS AND LOWER LEG

EXERCISE 10 Stand hands on hips, feet about 30 cm (12 in) apart, toes pointing almost straight to the front. Quick full knees bend and stretch, keeping the heels flat on the floor and back flat, not rounded.

It may be difficult at first to keep the heels on the floor when going into the knees bend position, so place two books under the heels, or use a small block of wood. A chair can be used for support in the early stages.

Breathe in just before the knees bend, out as you rise. Repeat twelve times. Rest and repeat again.

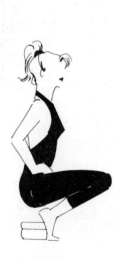

Exercise 10

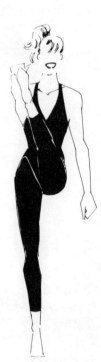

Exercise 11

EXERCISE 11 Stand hands at sides. Alternate leg swing forward, touching toes with opposite arm. Swing the leg as high as possible without bending the rear knee, and maintaining an upright position of the body.

34

Breathe normally. Repeat ten times with each leg. Rest and repeat again. Good progression can be made by swinging the leg forward and backward.

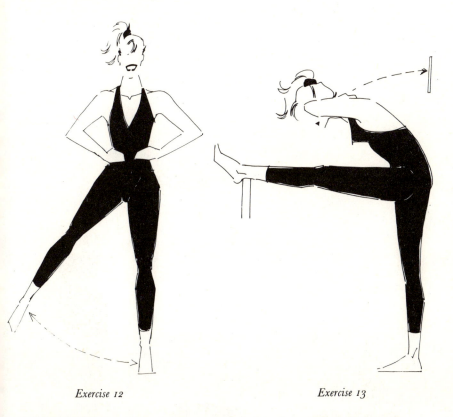

Exercise 12   *Exercise 13*

EXERCISE 12   Stand feet together, hands on hips. Swing leg sideways, as high as possible. Maintain an upright position. Breathe normally. Repeat ten times, then do the same with the other leg. Rest and repeat.

EXERCISE 13   Stand in neck rest position or hands on hips. Place one foot on a fairly high chair or table. Keep the rear leg straight and, bending the body forward, try to place the head on the outstretched leg.

At first you may only manage a slight forward bend. Do not worry, but ensure that both legs are straight. Repeat ten times, then change legs and repeat again. Breathe normally.

35

EXERCISES FOR THE TUMMY AND HIPS

These exercises are primarily to flatten the tummy and tone up and strengthen the muscles. But they also have a marked effect on the hips and thighs.

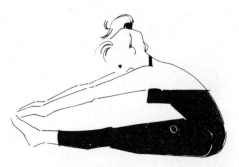

Exercise 14

EXERCISE 14 Lie on the floor, feet together, toes pointed, arms above the head. Anchor the feet under a chest of drawers, or get someone to hold the ankles. Swing the arms forward and sit up, reaching forward with the arms to touch the toes. Try to bend the body forward as far as possible.

This exercise may be difficult at first, so start in a sitting position, legs straight. Reach forward to touch the toes.

Try ten repetitions and later try the exercise from the lying position. Breathe normally.

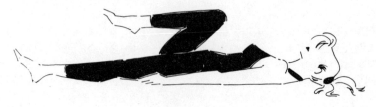

Exercise 15

EXERCISE 15 Lying on the back, hands at sides, legs straight and toes pointed. Alternate knee raise high to chest, keeping the other leg straight. Breathe normally. Repeat with the alternate leg until you have done ten repetitions with each leg. Rest and repeat again.

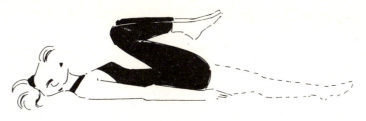

Exercise 16

EXERCISE 16   This is a progression of Exercise 15. Raise both knees together until they touch the chest. Make sure that the knees do not part. Breathe in as you raise the knees, breathe out as you lower them. Try ten repetitions. Later progress by doing two sets of ten repetitions.

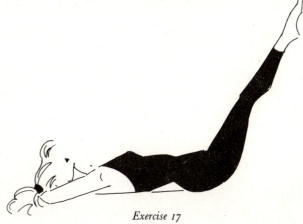

Exercise 17

EXERCISE 17   A further progression. Lie on the back, but adopt the neck rest position. Keeping the legs together and toes pointed, raise both legs 60 cm (2 ft) off the floor. Breathe in when raising the legs, out as you lower them. Repeat ten times. Rest and repeat another ten times.

This is a very advanced exercise. You will be getting really strong in the tummy when you can do ten repetitions correctly. You may at first only be able to do one or two repetitions. As you become more proficient, raise the legs higher, until you can put them right behind your head, touching the floor with your toes. But the legs must be kept straight.

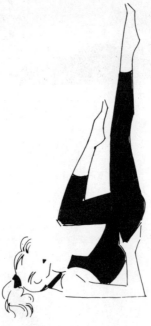

Exercise 18

EXERCISE 18   Finally, as an all-round tummy and hip exercise, try cycling. Lie on the back with high hip support. (This may take some practice, but I am assuming that you will be advanced when you try this.)

With the legs, perform a cycling movement, speeding up as you become proficient. Try to continue non-stop for approximately twenty seconds. Rest and repeat again. Breathe normally.

A progression on this exercise is done by keeping the legs straight and swinging them alternately forward and back to touch the toes of one foot on the floor behind the head.

EXERCISES FOR THE BACK

Many of the exercises already mentioned have a marked effect on the back, but one or two special ones for strengthening are essential in any exercise scheme for women.

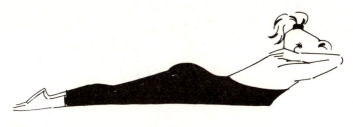

Exercise 19

EXERCISE 19   Lie face downwards, neck rest. Rest face on one side when in contact with the floor. Keeping the elbows well back, raise the head and chest as high as possible off the floor. Breathe in when lifting the head and chest, out when lowering the body. Turn the head to one side when on the floor to avoid breathing in dust.

This is a really strong back exercise. It may be wise to commence with the hands on the hips, progressing to the neck rest position later. Try ten repetitions. Rest and repeat.

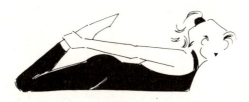

Exercise 20

EXERCISE 20   Lie face downwards as in Exercise 19. Grasp your ankles with your hands. Pull on the ankles and lift the head and chest as high as possible off the floor. Breathe in as you make the lift, out as you relax. Repeat ten times. Rest and repeat again.

This is an advanced exercise requiring suppleness in the back. Don't attempt it if you have to struggle.

Exercises 19 and 20 are also known as hyper extensions. They are strongly recommended as remedial exercises and for strengthening the back, but if you have any serious back problems diagnosed by your doctor, ask him to recommend a good physiotherapist to assist you if he suggests exercises. An eminent orthopaedic consultant advised me to remember that, in general, if you have backaches of any sort always remember to bend back rather than forward, to ease the pain. Hyper extensions are for this.

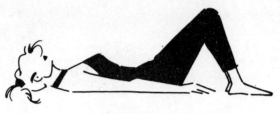

Exercise 21

EXERCISE 21 Breathing and Relaxation   Every training programme, whether freestanding work or weight training, should finish with this exercise. It restores the system to its normal tempo.

Lie on the back, arms at sides, palms of hands on floor. Raise the knees, keeping the soles of the feet on the floor. This will completely relax the tummy muscles and is an ideal resting position.

First, try to take all the hollows out of your back. Tuck your seat in and feel the whole of the spine flat against the floor. Breathe in slowly and completely through the nose. Then exhale very slowly and completely again through the nose. Repeat until you are completely rested and relaxed.

MAKING UP A TRAINING ROUTINE

An overall routine for a complete beginner can be made up by taking the first exercise in each group. Exercise 1 should in any case be done at the start of every workout. Then you go on with Exercise 2, Exercise 6, Exercise 10 (this should also be included in every workout), Exercise 11, Exercise 14 and Exercise 15 (same group), Exercise 19, Exercise 21 (also in every workout).

At first perform one set of repetitions of each exercise you select. Later you can progress to two sets of repetitions.

If you feel that you have a weakness in any particular part, such as posture, hips or tummy, select more than one exercise from each group to concentrate on the weakness.

You will note that I have selected two exercises from the 'hips, thighs and lower leg' group, and two from the 'tummy and hips' group. I feel this is very necessary for most women and that these are the parts where exercise is needed most.

Here is a more advanced routine. Exercise 1, Exercises 3 and 4,

Exercises 7 and 8, Exercises 10 and 12, Exercises 14 and 16, Exercise 19, Exercise 21.

A harder routine could consist of Exercise 1, Exercises 4 and 5, Exercises 8 and 9, Exercises 10, 12 and 13, Exercises 14 and 18, Exercise 20, Exercise 21.

Some of these exercises, particularly for the tummy, can be included in the weight training routine which is to follow in a later chapter.

Chapter 7

A BEAUTIFUL NECK FOR EVERY WOMAN

Woman are not as old as they used to be! At an age when their grandmothers had retired to the rocking-chair, today's women are still leading active lives. They have careers, and even enter dancing and beauty contests for glamorous grandmothers. And it is a courageous man indeed who will attempt to estimate a woman's age to within five years.

But some physical features are a cruel guide to age. One of the most accurate pointers is the condition of the neck. The first signs of age or ill health appear in this region. Have you noticed how many older women on TV or in public life try to hide their neck with clever fashions and even garments which will hide their neck?

You cannot always hide your neck, however. Modern styles of dress just don't allow it. So you must take special care to keep your neck young looking.

It can be done with the right exercises, though for some reason or other so many exercise plans forget about the neck altogether. It cannot be done by using cosmetics: they can hide age, up to a point, on the face, but they can do little for the neck.

The six exercises illustrated here and explained below will give you complete neck beauty. They will fill the hollows, smooth sagging skin and melt away double chins.

Try to do these exercises every day, if you feel that your neck needs special attention, but otherwise at least three times a week. They will so tone up the circulation that faded skin will be restored to normal colouring.

Many minor postural defects occur at the neck. These, too, will be improved by the exercises.

You may feel a little stiffness at first. But do not let this worry you. It is a sure sign that the muscles in the neck are weak and out of condition.

EXERCISE 1   Lie on the back on a table or bench. A bed or divan will do, but the exercises are more beneficial if done on a hard surface so that perfect position is maintained.

Let the head hang freely over the end of the bench. Raise the head as far as possible until the chin rests on the chest. Lower to starting position. Breathe normally. Repeat twelve times. Rest and repeat again.

Exercise 1

Exercise 2

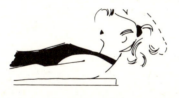

Exercise 3

EXERCISE 2   Lie sideways over the end of a table or bench; one shoulder and arm should also hang over the end. Let the head hang quite loosely sideways.

Raise the head sideways as high as possible, lower to starting position, and relax. Repeat twelve times, then turn on to other side for another twelve repetitions. Breathe normally.

EXERCISE 3   Lie at the end of table or bench, head hanging free. Rotate the head in a complete circle, first to the left, then to the right. Make the circles as big as possible and a complete movement. Repeat ten times in each direction.

43

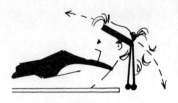

Exercise 4

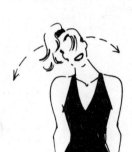

Exercise 5

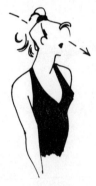

Exercise 6

EXERCISE 4   This is a repetition of Exercise 1, but resistance is added by tying a weight round the head. Headstraps specially for this exercise can be purchased, but they can easily be made with a disc weight attached to a band. Repeat ten times. Rest and repeat again. Breathe normally.

EXERCISE 5   Stand upright. Keeping the face to the front, move the head fairly rapidly from left to right. Repeat to count of twenty. Breathe normally.

EXERCISE 6   Stand upright. Circle the head first to the left, then to the right. Make a complete circle: forwards, sideways, backwards and sideways and to the front. Repeat ten times each way, starting to left and then to right.

Chapter 8

YOUR FEET NEED CARE

'My feet are killing me.' How often have you heard a friend say that? Many women seem to have come to expect aching feet almost as a birthright.

It is estimated that 5,000,000 women every year undergo foot treatment from chiropodists. This does not include women whose troubles are so acute that they need surgical and orthopaedic treatment.

It seems to be a fact that women are more prone to foot ailments than men. They spend more time on their feet, either in the house or at work, and they often wear shoes that are too small for them. Many are slaves to fashion or vanity, whatever the cost to their comfort and health.

Experts tell us that most foot troubles start back in our childhood, and ill-fitting shoes are often a primary cause. It is only in very recent years that manufacturers have started to give a wider range of between-sizes.

When a teenage girl leaves school she can go straight from solid, flat-heeled shoes into an exaggerated version of whatever happens to be the fashion of the day. Nobody is going to stop her. It's an inevitable sign of independence and growing up. And nobody is ever going to stop any woman from buying for fashion rather than for comfort and utility – at least, not until she is beyond caring.

I certainly don't intend to try it. I am going to content myself with suggesting that even fashionable shoes are more comfortable if they are the correct size. Take care of your feet, give them some strengthening exercises to offset bad posture, and you should be able to wear the latest creations without laying up too much future trouble for yourself.

Apart from any other consideration, poor feet are so ugly. I have seen many a dazzling beauty queen with dreadful feet when she has removed her shoes. The appearance of many otherwise well-groomed women is ruined by awful hard callouses at the backs of their heels, caused by ill-fitting and rubbing shoes.

Bunions, an enlargement of the bigger big toe joint, are common in both young and old. This condition is often self-inflicted by wearing the wrong shoes for years. It can be very painful and often has to be dealt with by a surgeon.

I need hardly say that feet cannot be washed too often. Afterwards, dry carefully and dust with talcum powder. Pay some attention to toe nails.

Feet must have air after being cooped up in shoes all day. Lack of air soon causes soreness. As often as you can, walk around the house in bare feet. Don't stand too long on cold or damp surfaces, of course.

After a hot bath plunge the feet into cold water. Then dry thoroughly, as always. The cold water will stimulate circulation and prevent chilblains and other skin ailments.

If you have bunions, corns or some other deformity, have them treated by a chiropodist. Make sure that your chiropodist is properly qualified (ask your doctor to recommend someone if you are in any doubt at all).

Ideally, of course, foot education should start at school. If you have young children make sure that they become foot conscious at an early age, and do teach them to walk correctly. When walking, the toes should point straight to the front. The foot should be placed on the ground in this sequence: heel, roll on to outer edge of foot, then toes.

You can practise this yourself in bare feet, maintaining proper posture. Exercise 1 in the freestanding group (page 29) makes a good combination postural and foot exercise.

One last point, before I list some special exercises for you to try. You may have flat feet. If your doctor had diagnosed this condition, and your feet do not hurt, there is unfortunately not much you can do to improve things. But if the muscles ache there is probably some simple weakness which can be strengthened and put right.

If your feet or ankles continually swell, consult your doctor, but if they do so only when tired, massage the ankles upwards, and rest by lying on the floor or a bed with the feet raised.

If you get itching splits between your toes you may have tinea or athlete's foot. This is a skin ailment which is very contagious. It needs medical attention. Good chemists have many medications for this condition, and also many other foot complaints. Do consult them if you have problems.

Now for those foot exercises. They are quite simple and you can do them in your room. Don't attempt the lot. Just select a few for each training session and vary them from time to time. Always do the exercises in bare feet.

EXERCISE 1   Commence by walking correctly round the room with toes to front. From there, walk on the toes for about thirty seconds, reaching as high as possible.

EXERCISE 2   Stand with feet about 15 cm (6 in) apart, toes to front. With a chair for balance, raise up on the toes and lower thirty times quickly. If you can place the toes on a block of wood about 8 cm (3 in) high, the exercise is more beneficial. Or a couple of firm books of identical height would do. If you perform this exercise with toes on a block of wood or on books, also force the heels towards the floor after raising up on them.

EXERCISE 3   Practise walking on the heels. Point the toes to the front, not out sideways. Try to do this for at least thirty seconds.

EXERCISE 4   Sit on a chair. Raise one foot off the floor, by crossing the legs if you wish. Rotate the ankle outwards, pointing the toes. Describe a complete circle outwards. Then do the same, rotating the ankle inwards. Do ten complete circles each way. Then change over to the other foot.

EXERCISE 5   Sit on a chair, feet flat on the floor, about 15 cm (6 in) apart, toes pointing to the front. Press the heels and pads of the toes on the floor and try to arch the insteps. This may give you a slight cramp at first, but it will strengthen the arches of the foot. Repeat twenty times.

EXERCISE 6   Stand with feet about 15 cm (6 in) apart, toes pointing to the front. Use a chair or piece of furniture for support. Rock forwards on the toes and back on to the heels. Lift the toes off the floor as high as they will go when rocking back. Repeat twenty times. Maintain upright posture.

EXERCISE 7   Sit with feet about 15 cm (6 in) apart. Slowly rub the sole of one foot up the shin of the other leg, and then down again. Repeat ten times with each foot.

EXERCISE 8   Sit with feet flat on floor, about 15 cm (6 in) apart, toes pointing to the front. Lift toes only off the floor, and then try to spread them outwards. Repeat ten times each foot.

EXERCISE 9   Sit with feet flat on floor, 15 cm (6 in) apart, toes to front. Screw up some little balls of paper, then try to pick them up off the floor with the soles of the feet. Repeat several times.

EXERCISE 10   Sit with one leg across the knee. Grasp the heel with one hand and the upper part of the foot firmly with the other. Twist the upper part of the foot upwards so you can see the sole of the foot (as if you were wringing it out). Hold the heel stationary. Repeat ten times slowly with each foot.

EXERCISE 11   Sitting, alternate ankle shaking with foot completely relaxed. Try to do this fast for thirty seconds with each foot.

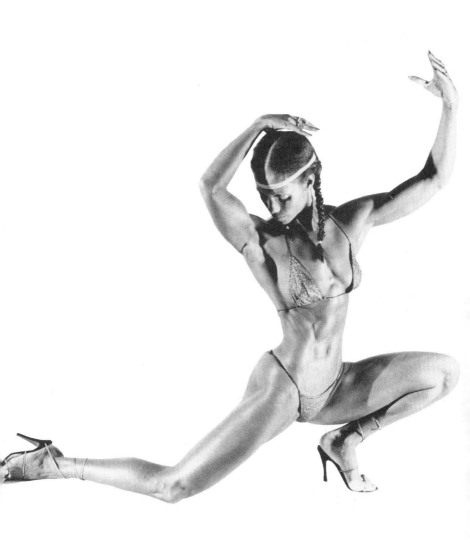

Jacqueline Nubret is typical of the modern concept of the perfect figure, slightly muscular, yet essentially feminine. She is an instructress at an international health club in Paris, has won international titles in physique contests, and has done top fashion modelling.

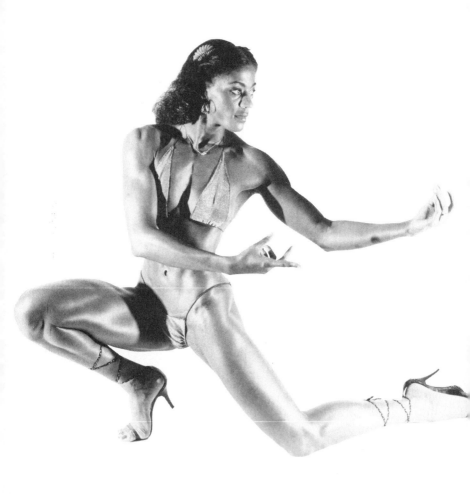

Jocelyne Pigsonneau, an international physique contest winner from Paris, displays her beautifully trained figure. She instructs at a health club and is a top fashion model.

Chapter 9

RESISTANCE EXERCISES USING HOUSEHOLD OBJECTS

In Chapter 6 I gave you twenty exercises which could be performed at home without using any apparatus or equipment. I hope that by now you have tried some of them for yourself and found them not so difficult at all.

I know many single women must exercise in bed-sitting rooms where there is not much space to move and where they cannot make a lot of noise. It is surprising, though, how much can be done in a small room, and certainly none of these exercises should disturb your neighbours.

Several times in previous pages I have mentioned weight training movements, resistance exercises using light dumbells and barbells, but before we attempt them, let us have a go at a half-way stage. Many simple freestanding exercises can be performed with added resistance to maintain progression merely by using ordinary objects found around the house.

Books, broomsticks and armchairs can be used as improvised equipment. Here are some suggestions which will lend added interest to your freestanding exercises and also help you to progress a stage farther along the road to health and beauty.

CHAIRS

You may have an armchair in your room, though a plain wooden chair will do.

Place your hands on the two arms of the chair and stretch your feet out behind you. Support the weight of the body on the arms. Bend the arms, lowering the chest towards the chair seat, and stretch.

This is called 'dipping'. It is a good shoulder and arm exercise. Of course, there are much harder versions of it, but if you can manage eight repetitions you are doing well. When you can do eight comfortably, rest, and do another eight repetitions.

BOOKS

Heavy books can be used to provide resistance for a great many exercises. I have already given you two good exercises with a book in Chapter 6 on freestanding work (Exercise 1, with the book on the head, and Exercise 5, pulling the book over to arms' length). Here are a few more you can do.

EXERCISE 1   Stand, holding a heavy book at the chest. Press the book overhead, reaching up as far as possible. Lower to the chest. Repeat ten times.

EXERCISE 2   Stand feet astride, holding a book above the head with both hands. Keeping the knees straight, swing the body forwards and downwards so that the book passes between the legs. Return to upright position and repeat ten times. The weight of the book will add quite a bit of resistance to the exercise, making it more effective than similar freestanding movements.

EXERCISE 3   Stand astride. Grasp a book above the head in both hands. Bend the body freely from side to side, but keeping the arms straight. Repeat to a count of twenty.

EXERCISE 4   Stand feet astride. Take a light book in each hand, arms at sides. Swing each book alternately or together overhead. Keep the body still. This is a fine exercise for moulding and lifting the bust.

EXERCISE 5   Stand feet astride. Hold a book in each hand, arms forward. Swing the arms sideways so that you feel the shoulder blades meet. Do not push the tummy forward. Repeat ten times. This is also a fine shoulder and bust exercise.

EXERCISE 6   Lie on the back, feet fixed under a chest of drawers or wardrobe, or with a friend holding them. Hold a book behind the neck, using both hands. Then sit up with it. This is the same as Exercise 14 in Chapter 6, but with added resistance.

BROOMSTICK

A broomstick can be used to add interest to many exercises.

EXERCISE 1   Stand feet astride. Hold the broomstick across the front of the thighs with both hands. The hands should be about shoulder-width apart. Swing the broomstick forwards and upwards above the head. Try to keep the body upright and confine the movement to the arms and shoulders. Repeat ten times.

EXERCISE 2   Stand feet well astride with a broomstick held across the back of the shoulders. Grasp the stick with the knuckles uppermost and use a fairly wide grip. Bend the body quite freely from side to side. Repeat twenty times.

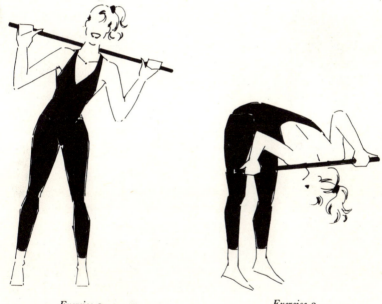

Exercise 2   *Exercise 3*

EXERCISE 3   The starting position is as for Exercise 2, with the broomstick behind the shoulders. Bend the body forward, keeping the knees straight. Do not force yourself at first. Keep the head back when bending forward so that the broomstick does not slip off your shoulders. Breathe in just before bending forward, breathe out as you return to the upright position.

EXERCISE 4   Stand as for Exercise 2 with the broomstick held across the back of the shoulders, with the feet about 46 cm (18 in) apart. Instead of bending from side to side, try twisting the body first to the left and then to the right as far as possible. Work from the waist only, trying to keep the hips square to the front and the feet fixed. You may not twist far at first, but you will improve as you get used to the exercise. Move the head freely and look behind you without moving the body. Breathe freely all the time.

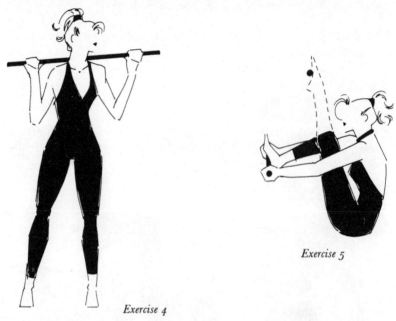

Exercise 5

Exercise 4

EXERCISE 5   Sit on the floor. Grasp the stick with hands about 60 cm (2 ft) apart. Raise one leg, bend the knee and put the sole of the foot against the stick between the hands. Holding on to the stick, straighten and bend the leg vigorously. Repeat.

EXERCISE 6   Stand with the feet astride, with the broom held in front of the thighs at arm's length, grip overgrip. Swing the broomstick forward and upward, keeping the arms straight all the time. Look straight ahead, do not follow the broomstick. Try not to bend backwards at all, but reach as tall as you possibly can without raising the heels. Breathe in as the broomstick moves forward and upwards, out as you return to the starting position.

EXERCISE 7 Lie on the back, arms straight behind the head, grasping the stick shoulder-width apart. Have the feet fixed or held unless you are strong in the tummy. Swing forward vigorously to sit up. Then reach forward with the stick as far as possible. Try to place your head on your knees. Try ten repetitions.

WRIST ROLLER

If you want to strengthen your wrists and forearms for tennis, this exercise is particularly useful. Many top-line sportswomen use it.

Tie a brick, flat iron or book to a piece of strong string. Wind the string round the centre of a piece of wood about 30 cm (1 ft) long and 4 or 5 cm (1½ or 2 in) in circumference.

Hold the stick with one hand at each end. Then, with the arms held out in front of you, wind and unwind the string to raise and lower the weight. Use only the wrists and forearms. You will soon find this tiring. As you progress, the weight can be increased.

BEACH BALL

You can devise any amount of exercises using a beach ball. Here are just four.

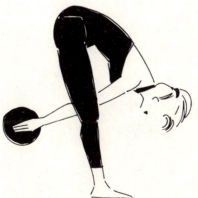

Exercise 1

EXERCISE 1 Stand feet astride, holding the ball in both hands with arms straight overhead. Swing the body forwards and downwards, reaching as far as possible between the legs. Return to upright position. Repeat ten times.

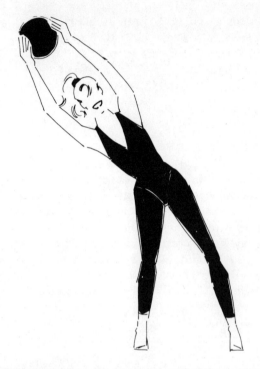

Exercises 2 and 3

EXERCISE 2   Same starting position as Exercise 1. Hold the ball overhead. Bend the body from side to side.

EXERCISE 3   Same as above, but describe a complete circle with the body, bending forwards, sideways and backwards.

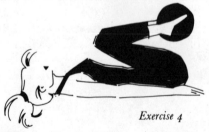

Exercise 4

EXERCISE 4   Lie on the floor, arms by your sides. Hold the ball between the feet. Raise the knees slowly to touch the chest, holding the ball between the feet. Lower to starting position. Breathe in just before you start to raise the knees to the chest, and out as you return to the starting position.

Chapter 10

OTHER APPARATUS

CHEST EXPANDERS

Most people have either seen or used a set of chest expanders. Chest expanders are sometimes called strands or cables. It is all the same thing. They are made of steel or rubber, or rubber covered with fabric. They have handles at either end so that the strands can be gripped and stretched across the chest.

Many women use expanders. They are not expensive, they are light to carry about and they do not take up any storage space.

The exercises for men and women are very similar, but, naturally, women do not need to use so much resistance. Most expander exercises are excellent for toning up the bust. Most expanders are sold with an exercise chart. Extra strands can always be bought separately for most good makes.

I suggest you use the rubber or fabric-covered type. Metal springs can sometimes pinch the skin when released, and they might catch your hair when performing exercises with the expanders near your head.

There are many excellent expander exercises for strengthening the muscles and maintaining mobility and suppleness for joints and ligaments. If you combine a few with some of the freestanding exercises I have already given, you will have a good, all-round training routine containing resistance work as well as bending and stretching.

I don't think you are likely to need the more elaborate expanders with various attachments, so I will concentrate on a few useful exercises for shoulders, arms, back, general posture and the upper body. You will appreciate, by the way, how the term 'chest expanders' came about. The best exercises with this equipment are for the upper body.

EXERCISE 1 SINGLE ARM FRONT CHEST PULL Stand astride, with one arm out sideways, holding the expander handle with the palm of the hand to the front. Hold the other handle across the chest, knuckles to the front. Keeping the arm already out sideways straight, pull the expanders across the chest with the other arm. You should finish up with both arms straight and the expanders across your chest. Repeat ten times. Then change arms and repeat once more.

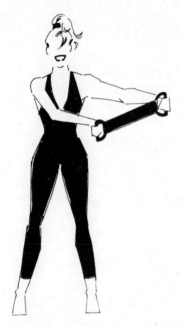

Exercise 1

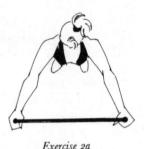

Exercise 2a

EXERCISE 2 TWO HANDS FRONT CHEST PULL This is a progression of the first exercise. Stand astride, holding the expanders with arms straight in front. Keeping the arms straight and with an even pull from both arms, pull the expanders across the front of the chest. The palms should be facing inwards when you grip the expanders. Repeat ten times. This is a fine bust, back and posture exercise. It can be done lying down on a bench, when it has an even better effect.

EXERCISE 3 OVERHEAD DOWNWARD PULL Stand astride, holding the expanders with arms straight above the head, palms of hands facing outwards. Keeping the arms straight, pull the expanders downwards across the back of the shoulders. It can

56

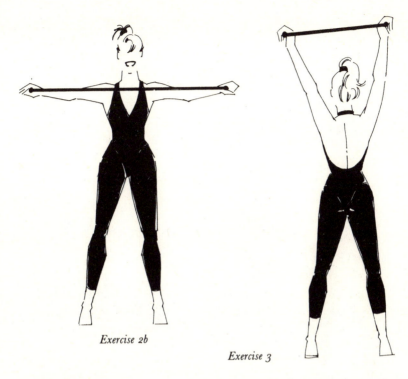

Exercise 2b

Exercise 3

be done by pulling the expanders downwards across the chest, but behind the neck is a better exercise. This is good for round shoulders, and for moulding the shoulders, back and backs of the arms. Repeat ten times.

EXERCISE 4 SINGLE ARM PRESS Stand feet astride. Hold the expanders with one hand close to the hip. With the expanders across the back, hold the other handle at the shoulder, palm of hand to the front. Keep the hand at the hip still and press the expanders overhead with the other hand. Repeat ten times. Then change over and do the same on the other side.

EXERCISE 5 BEND FORWARD FRONT CHEST PULL Stand astride with body bent forward, holding the expanders with knuckles outwards, arms in the hang position. Maintaining the forward bend position, pull the expanders across the chest. This is a fine bust and shoulder exercise. Repeat ten times.

57

The exercises above are the ones I consider best for women. But you can use expanders to combine with many freestanding exercises. Try sitting, alternate toe touch, with expanders held across the back, for instance.

When you are quite used to doing ten repetitions of each exercise, try a further set of ten repetitions. This is known as the 'set system'. It applies to all forms of exercise, whether freestanding, with expanders or with weights.

The ideal is to work up to three sets of eight or ten repetitions. Written, it is often expressed thus: 3 × 8.

A GYM BAR

Bars for hanging on, and for performing certain types of exercises for shoulders and tummy, are found in most modern gymnasiums. They are popular with women and sold in many big stores.

Men call this apparatus a 'chinning bar' because it is used mainly for doing 'pull-ups' of varying types. This form of exercise, though, is usually too strong for women. However, there are many other exercises which women can perform with a bar.

An extending bar can be purchased for fitting into any doorway, and is very useful. It can be put up or taken down in a matter of seconds, and it can be set at various heights for all sorts of exercises.

For many types of back strains, and for round shoulders and posture correction, hanging on a bar or beam at arms' length is a fine exercise in itself. The bar should, of course, be high enough for the arms to be straight and the feet clear of the floor.

When hanging on a bar of this type lift the chest up and force the heels right back. Hold the head high. This is an excellent exercise for women, and an all-round strengthener.

Here are some exercises which can be performed on a bar about 2.4 m (8 ft) from the floor:

EXERCISE 1   Hang on the bar, hands over the top. Keep the body braced. Swing from side to side; the movement coming from the hips and waist only. The upper body remains still. This is a great waist and lateral strengthening exercise.

EXERCISE 2   Hang as above, body firm. Raise alternate knees to chest. Try ten repetitions with each leg alternately.

EXERCISE 3   If you become really expert, you should be able to raise both knees at once, but that is a strong exercise.

By lowering the bar to about a metre (3 ft) off the floor, or slightly higher, you can do many exercises in a seated position, or in a hanging position with legs outstretched and hips off the floor.

IRON BOOTS OR BEAUTY BOOTS

For a start, don't be put off by the name 'iron boots'. They are a form of weight training equipment, and consist of metal over-shoes which are strapped over your exercise slippers.

The boots weigh about 2.7 kg (6 lb) each. You can make them heavier by attaching a short steel rod and small disc weights. Women like them particularly for waist, hips, thigh and lower leg exercises – all areas where you may wish to reduce or add to your measurements.

Plastic coated, lighter types are made specially for women, though you may have a man around the house who can improvise a pair for you.

If you look back to the freestanding exercises in Chapter 6, you will find that many of the leg, hip and waist exercises described can be performed while wearing iron boots. The exercises will become harder, of course, but they will be more progressive and you will definitely make quicker progress. Here are the exercises in Chapter 6 which can be performed wearing iron boots:

Legs and hips: Exercises 11 and 12.

Tummy: Exercises 15, 16, 17 and 18.

Go easy at first. Even a small amount of resistance in the form of weight adds considerably to the difficulty of the exercise. If you were able to do ten repetitions of the freestanding exercise you may well find that you can only manage two or three with the iron boots.

If this is the case, don't worry. Try to do three repetitions, then take a rest. Try again with further repetitions until you have repeated the exercise at least ten times. You will find Exercise 17 particularly hard.

Here are five special iron-boot exercises illustrated for you. They are for the lower legs, hips and thighs.

EXERCISE 1   Stand with your hands on your hips. Leg swing forwards and upwards. Repeat ten times each leg and gradually progress to twenty times. This is a fine exercise for the front of the thighs and hips.

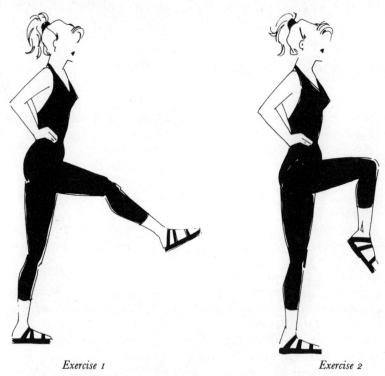

Exercise 1   *Exercise 2*

EXERCISE 2   Stand with your hands on your hips. Alternate knee raise high to chest. You should feel the pull on your hips and backs of the thighs. Repeat to count of twenty.

EXERCISE 3   Stand with your hands on your hips. Bending the knee, swing the lower leg backwards and upwards as far as possible. This is a good exercise for the calf of the leg and backs of the thighs. Repeat ten times each leg.

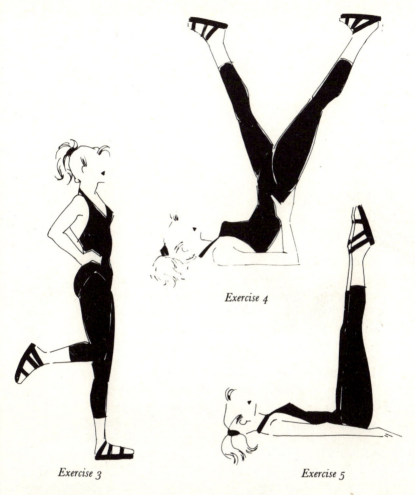

Exercise 4

Exercise 3

Exercise 5

EXERCISE 4   Lie on the back. Raise both legs to right angles, high hip support. Swing both legs sideways. This is a fine hip, inner thigh and tummy exercise. Do not be too vigorous at first. Repeat ten to twenty times.

EXERCISE 5   Lie on the back, hands at sides. Raise both legs together at right angles to the body. This is also described in the freestanding chapter. It is a very strong tummy and thigh exercise and should not be done until you are proficient. Work up to ten repetitions. Rest, and repeat.

EXERCISE 6 Sit on a table, legs hanging down normally. Straighten both legs together by extending the knees. Repeat fifteen times. This is good for hardening the front of the thighs and for strengthening knees after injuries.

EXERCISE 7 Stand with one hand on the back of a chair for support. Leg swing forwards as far as possible and then backwards, keeping body upright and both legs straight. This is a fine all-round hip and thigh exercise. Repeat ten to fifteen times with each leg.

THE VIBRATOR

All good gymnasiums, both for men and women, possess an electrically-operated vibrator. It is a wide, canvas belt which goes round the waist. The belt rotates round and round, or up and down, giving the mid-section a vigorous massage.

It can also be applied to hips, thighs and even arms, and is excellent for general toning up. They can be purchased for home use. The more sturdy type are best if you can afford them, the light ones wear out quickly if used regularly.

Vibrators are meant to tone up the muscles, and remove stiffness, help minor aches and pains, and stimulate the circulation. Far too many people imagine that a vibrator will melt away unwanted fat around the waist, hips and bottom. This is far from the truth, although they do tone up generally. It is no use going to a gym or even spending forty-five minutes at home reading a magazine with a vibrator round your bottom. I have often seen it done! Tone up with a vibrator before you start and when you finish your progressive exercises.

OTHER MULTI-PURPOSE EXERCISE MACHINES

Over the years many electrically-operated exercises have been put on the market. Most of them are expensive and no doubt the people who buy them find they are worth the money; personally I call them psychological exercises.

Of course, if you can use a health club or leisure centre for your exercises, you will find many new multi-purpose machines. The types are unlimited. Some are very cumbersome and very expensive. They can make training more interesting and more selective, and so prevent boredom. Some also save loading and unloading barbells and dumbells, to add or subtract the weight.

Basically, however, there is nothing that you cannot do with barbells and dumbells, a selection of discs of various poundages, and a bench. But, of course, this sort of exercise requires 'stickability' to get the results which are there if you make the effort.

There is no short cut to a good figure. It does require a little work and perseverence if you are to achieve results of which you will be proud. Some women are blessed with high potentiality, of course, and obtain quicker results than their less fortunate friends.

SUNLAMPS

Many health clubs now have sunlamps and sunbeds of various descriptions. There are many varieties from the simple table models to the new, expensive sunbeds.

I believe that the sunbeds really do tan, but you must take certain precautions, both to get the best out of effective treatment, but also to avoid those which are ineffective.

No one should undergo sunlamp treatment without consulting their medical advisor. They are not suitable for all types of skin, and can be very dangerous, especially if precautions are not taken to protect the eyes. In any case you can get severe burning, just like sunburn, without realising it, if you overdo it. People who have had certain types of illness, or skin problems, should most certainly consult their doctor who may recommend a dermatologist.

That does not mean to say that for those who are okay, and that is almost everyone, that they do not have a great deal of merit and make one feel good. But is is better to be safe than sorry.

Chapter 11

AN INTRODUCTION TO FIGURE TRAINING WITH WEIGHTS

In previous pages we have examined a variety of different exercises and several exercise techniques. We have looked at (and I hope tried) freestanding work. We have examined the possibilities of using household objects to obtain more resistance, and we have investigated various pieces of apparatus which will help us to exercise more easily and to make quicker progress.

Now I want to talk about the most flexible exercise method of all – weight training.

Let me repeat, once more, that weight training is now thoroughly respectable. It is accepted and encouraged by the various athletic bodies, and sportswomen everywhere practise it as a valuable aid to increased strength, stamina and muscular co-ordination. It is also excellent for weight reduction or building up weight, and for remedial purposes.

Every week, thousands of women (housewives, business girls and models) train with weights because they realise it is the finest way to keep a youthful figure and healthy good looks. Some of them exercise in gymnasiums, but many have to train at home.

So let me ask just one favour of you. Please firmly banish from your mind any pictures of huge musclemen staggering under the crushing weight of enormous barbells. You are not going to lift heavy weights. You are not going to develop big muscles.

Weight training will take off surplus weight, and it will also put on flesh where it is really needed. Correctly practised it will bring quick, sure results. I most strongly urge you to give it a fair and reasonable trial. You will never regret it, believe me.

There are literally hundreds of weight training exercises. If I gave only half of them you would end up by becoming thoroughly confused. I have therefore picked the ones I consider most useful for women in their pursuit of figure beauty and good health.

Most of these exercises are basic and are performed by both men and women. Many other exercises are specialised muscle-building work for men and obviously are not included.

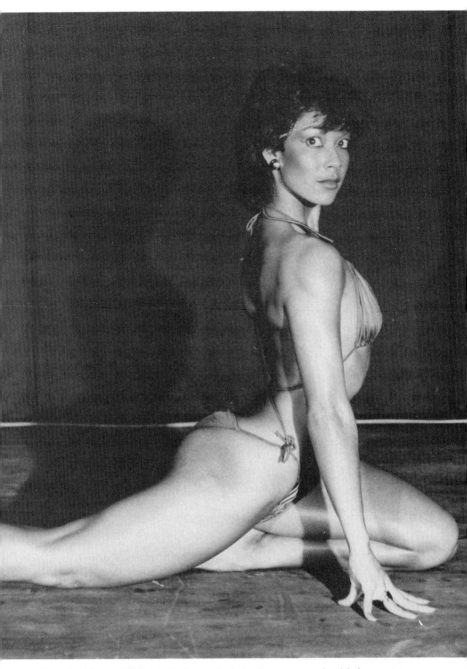

Elena Eeidelman of Holland. In the top physical culture contests, the girls have to pose in this way to show the flexibility and general grace of their figures. In other words, they have trained figures.

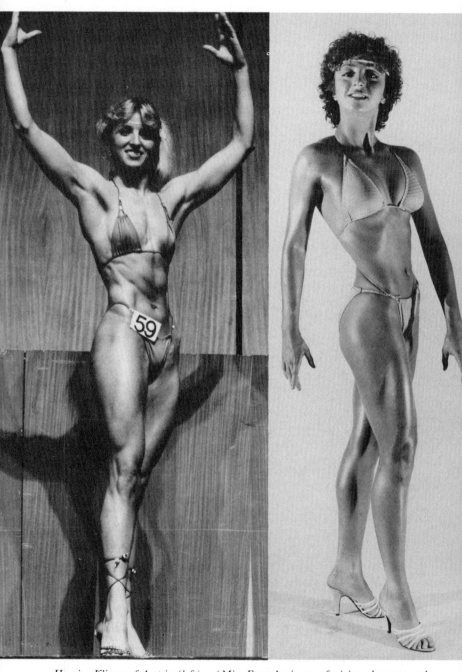

Hermine Klinger of Austria (left), a 'Miss Europe' winner – feminine, glamorous and a picture of good health.

On the right, my ideal modern woman – perfectly fit, with a well balanced figure, and entirely feminine. Ramos is Spanish. She combines weight training with dancing.

I sincerely hope you will attempt some weight training. It does not need much space and it is not going to make any noise.

EQUIPMENT

Basic weight training equipment is the barbell; a length of steel rod with cast-iron disc weights at either end.

For women, the steel rod (or bar) should not be more than 1.5 m (5 ft) long. A stock size is 1.4 m (4 ft 6 in), and this is ideal. It will weigh about 6.8 kg (15 lb) and have a diameter of 2.5 to 5 cm (1 to 1½ in). Some bars are covered with a chrome 'sleeve'; this makes the bar easier to handle and saves the hands.

If you buy a barbell set complete from a sports shop you will also get some short dumbell rods, weighing about 2.3 kg (5 lb) each including handles for gripping.

In many sports shops today you will find special women's barbell sets with shorter bars, but most women manage with men's equipment, just using shorter bars and lighter discs.

The actual weights are in the form of cast-iron discs, and they can weigh anything from 500 g to 22 kg (1¼ to 50 lb). They are secured to the bar or dumbell rods with metal 'collars' which either screw on or have patent quick-release fasteners. It is because the weights on a bar can be changed at will to give any required resistance that weight training is such a flexible and progressive exercise system.

Whenever you exercise, always make sure that the discs are secured to the bar with these collars. If you don't, the discs will slide, throwing you off balance. They could easily hurt you and, anyway, if they fall on the floor you will discover that weight training can be a noisy pastime after all.

By loading discs centrally on one of the dumbell rods you can make a swingbell. This is a most useful gadget for women and I will later be giving you some exercises for it. (As a matter of interest, 'dumbells' are so called because in the old days they were hollow metal balls filled with sand to give additional weight.)

The only other equipment you need is a bench. They are supplied in sports shops. They can be quite expensive, especially if they are hinged to make 'an incline bench', but a flat bench is adequate and should be a minimum of about a metre (3 ft) long, 38 to 46 cm (15 to 18 in) wide, and about 76 cm (2 ft 6 in) high. If you cannot afford a bench, they can be improvised with a plank of wood 1 m (3 ft) long by 30 to 45 cm (1 to 1 ft 6 in) wide. It should be supported off the ground so that your feet reach the floor comfortably when lying on your back on the bench. It should also be padded, or covered with a blanket or piece of felt, so that the wood does not cut into your back and shoulders. There is no need to be uncomfortable while exercising.

Weight training equipment is not cheap, but it never breaks and will last a lifetime. You can buy more metal discs to increase resistance as and when you require them.

If you are going to buy a packaged set I suggest one weighing about 22 kg (50 lb) in all. Make sure that you get a good variety of the lighter discs, rather than a couple of the big ones weighing 7 kg (15 lb) or more each, and which you will seldom, if ever, need.

As I have said, the bar alone weighs about 7 kg (15 lb), and the dumbell rods around 2.3 kg (5 lb) each. For a beginner this is all that will be needed when starting on a lot of exercises. If you find a steel bar hurts your hands, wear an old pair of gloves made of some material that is not going to slip.

A TRAINING SESSION

How long should a training period last? It can be fifteen to twenty minutes. It can be well over an hour. But unless you are a trained athlete anything over one hour is not recommended.

Remember that weight training is just about the most concentrated form of exercise known. In fifteen minutes you can do more exercise, and bring more major muscle groups into play, than in an hour's freestanding work or in two hours of games.

To some extent games tend to cause one-sided development. (Some athletes train to counteract this tendency.) But weight training exercises every part of the body evenly, and yet still allows you to concentrate on specific parts which need special attention, or where there is a weakness.

You should start every training period with one or two freestanding exercises (described and illustrated in Chapter 6). These loosen your joints and prepare the system for tougher work.

Every session should also include tummy and waist exercises – do them at the beginning or the end. You can do tummy exercises with weights, but I believe they are too strenuous for women.

66

Once you have started on the weight training road to figure beauty, try to workout at least twice a week, and three times a week if you can possibly manage it. Be sure to have a complete day of rest between each session, though you can do a few freestanding exercises if you like. The rest day is most important. It allows your muscles to relax and repair themselves.

THE SET SYSTEM

I briefly mentioned the set system in an earlier chapter, but I must now explain it in greater detail as it affects weight training. It is the most widely used modern technique, and the best one, both for figure training and for athletic improvement.

You can perform each exercise, repeating it without a break for a 'set' of several repetitions (eight or ten is the usual number). Then you can have a short rest and perform another set, and so on. The rest is only long enough to allow breathing to return to normal. A longer rest between sets ruins the continuity of the training session.

Most people perform three sets of an exercise. But you can vary this number with experience and to suit your own training needs.

When you have completed the required number of sets for one exercise, you go on to the next exercise on your list. The set system enables you to concentrate on one particular area of the body before proceeding to another. Blood is drawn to the exercise area and helps to strengthen and mould the tissue.

Three sets of ten repetitions means that you perform thirty repetitions in all, with a short breather after each ten repetitions. A beginner will start with one set only, and progress to three as strength increases.

Women who want to reduce should perform high repetitions, i.e. three sets of up to fifteen repetitions. And women who want to put on weight should perform low repetitions, i.e. three sets of five or six, but with more weight.

Naturally, if you are working on high repetitions you will use a lighter weight, and if you are attempting low repetitions you will use a heavier weight, so the total amount of work performed is going to be the same.

WHAT WEIGHTS TO USE

How much weight should you use for each exercise? It is a difficult question. So much depends on the individual; on age, bodyweight, strength and potentiality.

It may take you a few training sessions to find out your own capabilities, but I advise you to start with very light weights. Ensure, above all, that you are doing each exercise correctly and with a full range of movement. It is also most important that you breathe correctly during each exercise.

A given weight may seem light enough after the first repetition, but it may need quite an effort to squeeze out the last three repetitions.

After you have got used to handling the barbell, and can perform an exercise correctly for a few repetitions, you will find it gratifyingly easy to add 2.3 kg (5 lb) or more to the weight used. This does not necessarily mean that you are getting stronger; it does mean that you are getting used to the exercise. Only when you can perform an exercise quite easily should you add further weight to the barbell or dumbell.

The human body is a complex machine. You can take two women, with identical measurements and bodyweight and one will be stronger on a certain exercise than the other. It depends on varying physical structure: leverages, bone lengths, centre of gravity and things like that. But this is really a theme for a work on physiology, not figure beauty. Temperament plays a very big part in success or failure, as it does in success or failure in diet.

Once you have decided on a certain routine of exercises, stick to it for eight to ten weeks before making a change. I am assuming now that you will be training three times a week. Anyway, about twenty-five to thirty sessions in all on the same routine is about right. Even then, some of the basic movements will remain.

Whatever you do, don't constantly chop and change from one routine to another. You will be doomed to failure. Women tend to try this with diets and exercise systems they read about in magazines. It is fatal.

There are certain advantages in training with a partner, or in a small group of friends, either at home or in a club. A little competition is a great incentive to effort, and some of the exercises do need a helping hand to get the weights into position.

Let me reassure you on one point that may worry you after your

68

first training session. Of course, you are going to feel stiff at first. Don't let it alarm you in any way. You have not done yourself the slightest harm. Finish with some freestanding limbering exercises, observe your rest day, and then continue the routine. The stiffness will soon be a thing of the past.

Soon, you will begin to feel stronger. You will become more confident in your movements. Your limbs will grow firm and moulded, and curves will begin to appear in the right places. Then you will know the real meaning of feeling fit.

If you are a heavy smoker I guarantee that you will be buying fewer cigarettes after the first weeks of training. After all, smoking is mainly a soother for jangled nerves. Your new-found fitness will help your nerves and reduce the need for constant smoking.

In the next chapter I am going to tell you about the best exercises for weight training. I shall describe them in detail, with illustrations.

I shall suggest starting weights suitable for an average beginner who is reasonably healthy and of average height and weight. These will only be a guide. Don't worry if you find you have to use less weight, and don't be too elated if you find you can manage more. I cannot assess your potential; I can only help you to find that out for yourself.

Finally, I shall make up some typical routines for you. They will incorporate some of the freestanding work in Chapter 6 and perhaps one or two of the iron-boot exercises.

Chapter 12

BASIC WEIGHT TRAINING AT HOME OR IN A GYM

I have already told you something about the various types of weight training appliances you are likely to need, the weights of the bars, dumbells, and so on.

In this chapter I will describe some of the many weight training exercises I recommend as most suitable for women. Every exercise is illustrated and I hope you will study the illustrations first so that when you read the description it will not seem quite so strange to you.

CHECKLIST OF EXERCISES

BARBELL EXERCISES – UPPER BODY
1. The Clean (correct method of lifting bar off floor)
2. Seated Press
3. Press Behind Neck
4. Straight Arm Pullover
5. Bench Press
6. Upright Rowing
7. Bent Over Rowing
8. Good Morning Exercise
9. Stiff-Legged Dead Lift
10. Curl

DUMBELL EXERCISES – UPPER BODY
11. Alternate Dumbell Press Standing
12. Alternate Dumbell Press Seated
13. Sidebends
14. Flying
15. Lateral Raise Sideways

SWINGBELL AND DISC EXERCISES – UPPER BODY
16. Straight Arm Pullover

17. Lateral Raise Lying
18. Swingbell Swing

BARBELL EXERCISES – THIGHS, LOWER LEGS, HIPS
19. Squat
20. Front Squat
21. Forward Lunge
22. Heels Raise Bar Across Shoulders and Upward Jumps
23. Heels Raise Bar Across Hips
24. Heels Raise Bar in Front of Thighs
25. Seated Heels Raise

DUMBELL EXERCISES – THIGHS, LOWER LEGS, HIPS
26. Squat
27. Jumping Squat
28. Leg Curl Machine

TUMMY EXERCISES
29. Sit up with Disc behind Head

You may be a little bit puzzled at first about how to grip the bar, how far apart your hands should be placed, and so on.

In most exercises the hands are placed about shoulder-width apart, and care must be taken to ensure that the bar is balanced before lifting it off the floor, that means the distances from each end of the bar to the hands are equal. Some people need a wider grip than others; a great deal depends on your build, and the length of your arms.

Where I state 'narrow grip' the hands should not be more than 30 cm (1 ft) apart, but for most exercises the distance between the hands should be between 45 and 60 cm (1 ft 6 in and 2 ft).

The terms 'overgrip' and 'undergrip' may be new to you. Overgrip is when the hands are placed over the top of the bar, knuckles uppermost, and thumbs under the bar. The thumbs should always grip round the bar for safety. Undergrip is when you grip the bar underneath, with the palms of the hands facing upwards, thumbs gripping round the bar as for overgrip.

Here then is a detailed description of all your exercises.

BARBELL EXERCISES FOR THE UPPER BODY

First things first. It is most important that you learn how to pick up a barbell correctly from the floor to the shoulders. This is the commencing position of many of the exercises, and it is also a fine exercise in itself.

The action of lifting the loaded barbell from the floor to the chest is called the 'Clean'. The whole exercise is known as 'cleaning the bar to the shoulders'.

EXERCISE 1 THE CLEAN   Stand with legs slightly astride, feet about 38 cm (15 in) apart, insteps against the bar and toes pointing to the front. Bend the knees, keeping the back quite flat and holding the head and chest well up. Grasp the bar with both hands, so that the thumbs are underneath and the knuckles on top. The hands should be slightly more than shoulder-width apart.

In this initial position, with the knees bent and the seat near the floor, the arms must be kept straight and the heels flat on the floor. Then sink back on the heels, and with a vigorous pull of the arms, pull the bar upwards towards the chest. When the bar is as high as possible, twist the wrists quickly and pull the bar into position, holding it high against the neck. Elbows must be kept well up, and the weight resting mostly on the ball part of the thumbs.

The lift must be fast and one continuous movement. The back and legs do most of the work. This exercise may need quite a bit of practice, and calls for balance and co-ordination.

Breathe in just before making the lift, out as the bar reaches the shoulders. I suggest 11 kg (25 lb) to commence.

EXERCISE 2 STANDING PRESS   Standing with the feet astride, pull the bar to the chest, as above. Press the bar overhead, passing it as near to the face as possible. Reach up high, but do not raise the head to look at the bar. Keep the head looking straight to the front. Breathe in just before pressing the bar overhead, and out as the bar is lowered to the chest.

This exercise can be done in a seated position, but is more advanced. It has its merits as once seated on a bench, you can maintain better posture. If you bend backwards at all you will overbalance. Remember this when performing the standing press; concentrate on not leaning back as you press the bar overhead. This is a fine shoulder and back exercise. Start with 6.8 kg (15 lb).

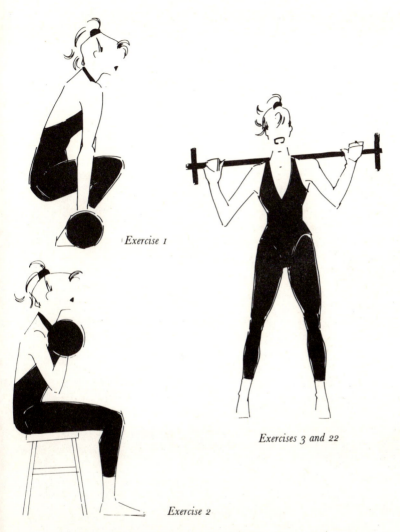

Exercise 1

Exercises 3 and 22

Exercise 2

EXERCISE 3 PRESS BEHIND NECK   After cleaning the bar to the chest, press it overhead, but on the way down lower it to the back of the neck, instead of to the chest.

Continue to press from the behind neck position. Let the bar touch the back of the neck each time. Breathe in just before making the press, out as you lower the weight to the neck.

This is a fine posture exercise and good for shoulders, back, chest and arms. Try 6.8 kg (15 lb) to commence.

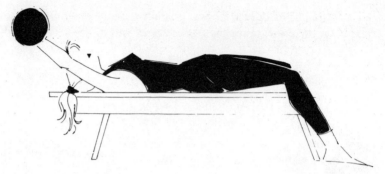

Exercise 4

EXERCISE 4 STRAIGHT ARM PULLOVER Lie on a bench, feet flat on the floor on either side of the bench. Hold a light bar above the head, palms of hands to front and with a fairly wide grip. Keeping the arms straight, lower the bar until the arms are outstretched behind the head. Raise the bar again to starting position and repeat.

Breathe in as the bar is lowered behind the head, out as the bar is returned to starting position. Do not take the bar behind the head beyond the normal stretch of the shoulder girdle.

This is a fine exercise for the shoulders, rib box and chest. It is widely used as a posture correction exercise, and also as an assistance exercise for all forms of sport. Try 4.5 kg (10 lb) to commence. A 'swingbell' (centrally loaded dumbell rod) is useful for this exercise.

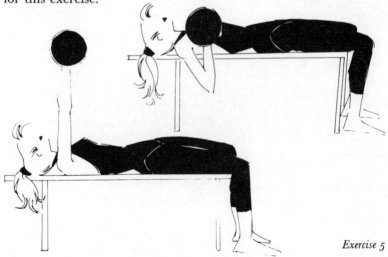

Exercise 5

EXERCISE 5 BENCH PRESS   Lie on a bench, feet either side and flat on the floor. Hold the bar at arms' length above the head, hands slightly wider than shoulder-width apart. If possible, the bar should be handed to you by a partner.

Lower the bar to the chest, and press it overhead. Breathe in while the bar is lowered to the chest, out as the press to overhead position is completed. This is one of the best general exercises for the bust and chest.

Ensure that the hips do not lift off the bench at any time during the exercise; this is important. Try 13.6 kg (30 lb) to commence.

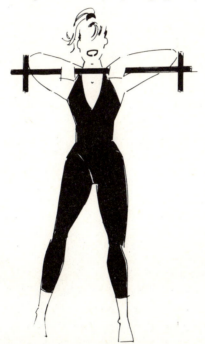

Exercise 6

EXERCISE 6 UPRIGHT ROWING   Stand with feet about 38 cm (15 in) apart, toes to front. Hold the bar in the hang position, arms straight, hands about 10 cm (4 in) apart, knuckles to the front. Pull the bar upwards by bending the elbows and raising them as high as you can. Keep the bar as close to the body as possible until it touches the chin. Lower to starting position and repeat.

Breathe in as the upward pull is made, out as the bar is lowered. This is a fine arm, shoulder and bust exercise. Try 9 kg (20 lb).

75

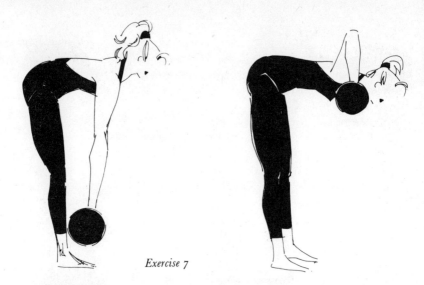

Exercise 7

EXERCISE 7 BENT OVER ROWING   Stand with legs fairly well astride, toes pointing to the front. Keep the legs straight and bend forwards until the body is at right angles to the legs. With the back straight and the arms in the hang position, grasp the bar, knuckles uppermost and hands slightly wider than shoulder-width apart. Pull the bar up to the chest without body movement.

Breathe in as the pull is made, out as the bar is lowered to starting position. This is a fine upper back and arm exercise, and also a stamina builder. Try 9 kg (20 lb) to commence.

EXERCISE 8 GOOD MORNING EXERCISE   Stand with feet astride, toes to front, bar behind the neck across the shoulders. Keeping the head well back, so that the bar does not roll off the neck, bend the body forwards slowly until it is at right angles to the legs. Return to upright position.

Breathe out as the body is lowered, in as you return to the upright position. This is a great lower back and posture exercise. It also stretches the long tendons at the backs of the legs, so compensating for the shortening created by the constant wearing of high heels. Commence with 6.8 kg (15 lb).

A slight knee bend is allowable for Exercises 7 and 8 to avoid any strain, but when well advanced, the legs should be kept straight.

EXERCISE 9 STIFF-LEGGED DEAD LIFT   Stand with feet together or about 30 cm (1 ft) apart. Grasp the bar overgrip, hands about shoulder-width apart. Lower the bar to the floor, keeping it

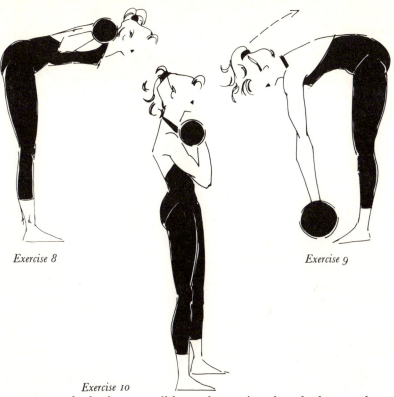

Exercise 8

Exercise 9

Exercise 10

as near to the body as possible, and ensuring that the legs are kept straight. As soon as the discs touch the floor, return to the upright position. Breathe in as you lift the bar, out as you lower it. When the lift is completed brace the shoulders back and lift the chest up.

This is a fine exercise for strengthening the whole of the back. It should only be practised when some general experience has been gained. Try 13.6 kg (30 lb) to commence.

EXERCISE 10 THE CURL   This exercise has many variations and can also be performed with a swingbell. It is an all-round arm and wrist exercise, ideal for trimming down or building up.

Stand with legs slightly astride. Hold a barbell at the hang position across the thighs, palms of hands to the front (undergrip), and about shoulder-width apart.

Without any body movement 'curl' and bar upwards to the shoulders by raising the arms from the elbows. Lift the elbows well up. Breathe in as the Curl is made, out as you lower the bar. Ensure that the bar is lowered to full stretch of the elbows. The initial pull is most important in this exercise. Try 9 kg (20 lb) to commence.

DUMBELL EXERCISES – UPPER BODY

EXERCISE 11 ALTERNATE DUMBELL PRESS   Stand with legs slightly astride. Lift two dumbells off the floor in the manner described for the Clean (Exercise 1). Keeping the body straight, press the right dumbell overhead with a vigorous thrust. Then lower it to the shoulder, simultaneously pressing the left dumbell overhead. Keep the dumbells as close together as possible; it will help you to maintain your balance.

    Try to get a rhythm with the exercise. Breathe freely. This is a fine shoulder, back and chest exercise. Try two 2.3 kg (5 lb) dumbells to commence.

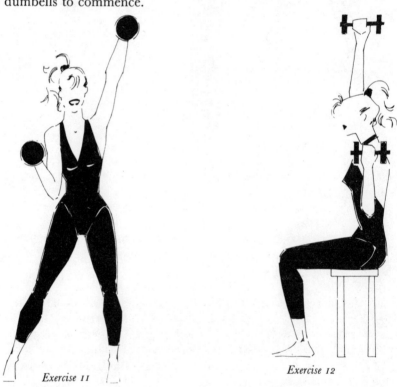

Exercise 11

Exercise 12

EXERCISE 12 ALTERNATE DUMBELL PRESS SEATED   This is a progression of Exercise 11. It requires perfect position of the body and more balance, and is a tougher exercise. A further advance is to press both the dumbells together overhead. Commence with the same weight as Exercise 11.

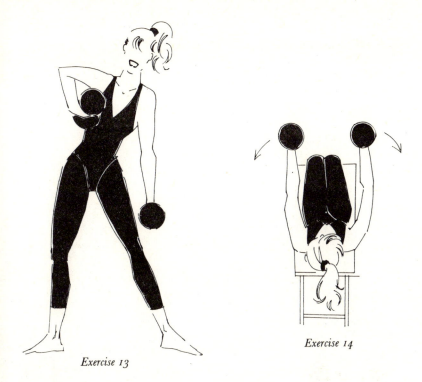

Exercise 14

Exercise 13

EXERCISE 13 SIDEBEND   Stand with legs astride, holding a dumbell in each hand. Trunk bend from side to side freely, with head and neck relaxed. As you bend, pull the opposite dumbell as far as you can up your side. The body must be kept straight with no forwards or backwards lean. Try to do the exercise rhythmically. Breathe freely. A 2.3 kg (5 lb) dumbell in each hand will be sufficient.

EXERCISE 14 FLYING EXERCISE   Lie on a bench, feet flat on the floor either side of the bench. Hold a dumbell overhead in each hand. Lower the dumbells outwards by bending the arms until they are below the level of the chest. Return to overhead position, arms above head. The starting position is the same as for Bench Press (Exercise 5).

   As you progress, the arms can be taken out wider and sideways until almost straight. Care must be taken not to straighten the elbows completely. Breathe in as the dumbells are lowered, out as you return to overhead position. Two 2.3 kg (5 lb) dumbells to commence.

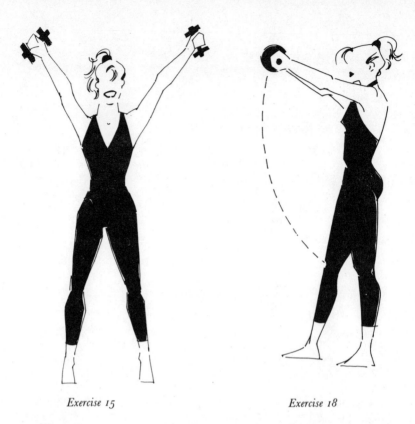

Exercise 15   *Exercise 18*

EXERCISE 15 LATERAL RAISE SIDEWAYS AND UPWARDS Stand with legs astride, a dumbell in each hand, arms at the hang position. Keeping the arms straight and the body erect, raise the dumbells out sideways as high as possible. Lower to starting position.

Breathe in as the dumbells are raised, out as you lower them. This is a fine shoulder and back exercise, and also generally lifts and tones the rib box. Try two 2.3 kg (5 lb) dumbells for a start.

SWINGBELL OR LIGHT DISC ONLY EXERCISES – UPPER BODY

EXERCISE 16 STRAIGHT ARM PULLOVER WITH SWINGBELL This is the same as Exercise 4 already described. A swingbell may be easier for a beginner. Commence with 6.8 kg (15 lb).

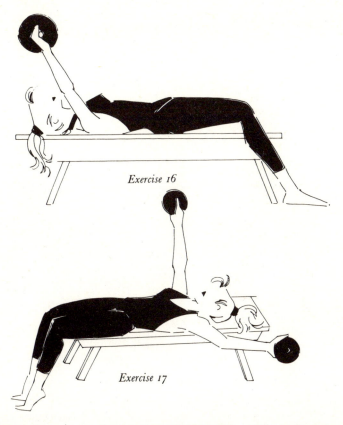

Exercise 16

Exercise 17

EXERCISE 17 LATERAL RAISE LYING   This is the same as
Exercise 14, Flying, but the arms are kept straight, and the weight
taken out sideways. It is a difficult exercise and two lights discs only
should be sufficient. Later, it can be tried with light dumbells. I
suggest two 2.3 kg (5 lb) discs to commence.

EXERCISE 18 SWINGBELL SWINGS   Stand with legs well
astride, trunk in the forward bend position. Hold a swingbell in
both hands. Keeping the legs straight, swing the weight upwards,
straightening the trunk. Return only to the upright position, but
later continue by swinging the weight until the arms are straight
above the head. This may require a little balance at first.

Breathe in on the upward swing, out as the forward bend is
made. This is a fine back, shoulder and waist exercise. Commence
with a 4.5 kg (10 lb) swingbell.

BARBELL EXERCISES – THIGHS, LOWER LEGS, HIPS

EXERCISE 19 THE SQUAT OR KNEES BEND Besides being a fine exercise for the thighs and back, the Squat is a great builder of stamina, and it will improve lung power and generally strengthen the chest and breathing system. It should be included in every training routine in some form. It is particularly good for athletes and sportswomen.

Stand with legs slightly astride, toes pointing to the front. With a barbell held across the shoulders behind the neck, bend the knees and sink into a knees bend position. Immediately return to the upright position.

Breathe in very deeply just before bending the knees, out as you return to the upright position. It is a good thing to breathe in and out a couple of times before each repetition. This will add to the benefit of the exercise.

The back must be kept flat – this is very important. If there is any sag or lack of control you may strain your back. Do not attempt to make a full knees bend unless you are supple in the hips; thighs slightly below the horizontal is sufficient.

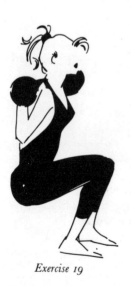

Exercise 19

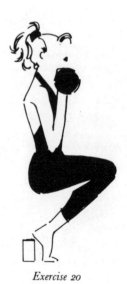

Exercise 20

The heels must be kept flat on the floor all the time. You may find this difficult. If there is a tendency for the heels to leave the floor as you bend the knees, put a book or block of wood about 5 to 8 cm (2 to 3 in) high under the heels.

Try 11 kg (25 lb) for a start. Pad your neck with a towel if the bar hurts it.

EXERCISE 20   THE FRONT SQUAT   This is exactly the same as the previous exercise, but this time the weight is held at the neck in the Clean position instead of across the shoulders. It is a harder exercise and requires better balance. It also gives more exercise to the front of the thighs. Commence with 9 kg (20 lb).

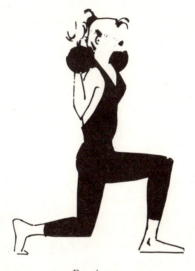

Exercise 21

EXERCISE 21 THE FORWARD LUNGE   With the bar held across the back of the shoulders, as explained for Exercise 19, step forward deeply with the right leg so that the lower leg is at right angles to the thigh. Bend the rear knee.

The deeper you can lunge the more benefit will be derived by the thighs and hips, but be cautious at first. Return to starting position and repeat the exercise with alternate leg lunging forward. The body must be kept upright all the time. Breathe in as the lunge is made, out as you return. Try 9 kg (20 lb).

83

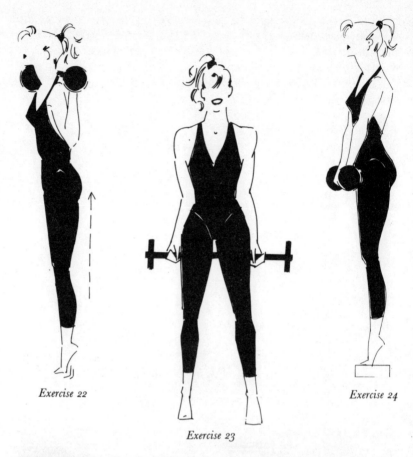

Exercise 22

Exercise 24

Exercise 23

EXERCISES 22, 23, 24 HEELS RAISE WITH BAR ACROSS SHOULDERS, ACROSS HIPS OR ACROSS FRONT OF THIGHS   These three exercises are all the same, except that the bar is held in different positions. In this way, the weight may be thrown onto slightly different parts of the muscles of the lower leg. They are all exercises for moulding and shaping the lower leg.

Stand with legs slightly astride, toes pointing straight to the front, bar held in both hands. Raise up on the toes as high as you can, hold the position, if possible, for a second or two and lower heels. You will find you can perform quite high repetitions with these three exercises. Try an 11 kg (25 lb) barbell to start. With bar across shoulders, upward jumps can also be included as a fine exercise for athletes and sportswomen.

EXERCISE 25 SEATED HEELS RAISE   Sit on a stool or chair
with a barbell resting across the knees and the toes supported on a
block of wood or some books. Raise the heels as high as possible and
lower. This is a very fine exercise for shaping or reducing the lower
leg. It should be performed with high repetitions. Try a 13.6 kg
(30 lb) barbell to start. Pad the knees with a folded towel if
necessary.

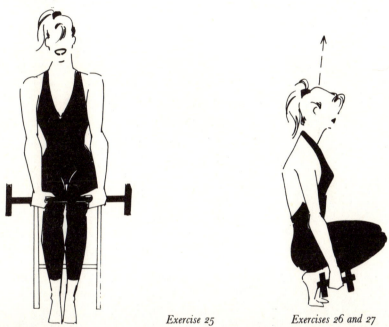

Exercise 25   *Exercises 26 and 27*

DUMBELL EXERCISES – THIGHS, LOWER LEGS, HIPS

**EXERCISES 26 AND 27 SQUATS OR JUMPING
SQUATS**   These exercises are performed in the same way as
Exercise 19, but a dumbell is held in each hand instead of a barbell.
Arms are kept at the hang position. See Exercise 19 for full details.

As a progression, and particularly for athletes and sportswomen,
the Squat can be performed with an upward jump, coming down
into the knees bend position. Naturally, a much lighter weight
should be used.

For ordinary Squats, try two 4.5 kg (10 lb) dumbells. For
Jumping Squats, two 2.3 kg (5 lb) dumbells.

85

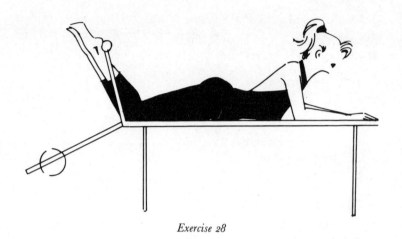

Exercise 28

EXERCISE 28 LEG CURL MACHINE   You may find this piece of equipment in a well-equipped gym, but it is a luxury. By curling the back of the heels under a bar, and pulling on a weight, the backs of the thighs and buttocks can be exercised. In a seated position the machine can also be used to exercise the front of the thighs. It is illustrated to show the scope of weight training appliances.

Thigh extension machines are also commonly used. Sitting upright with the legs outstretched and the insteps under a weighted bar, pull the bar towards you and then drop it back to the starting position.

TUMMY EXERCISES

Except for trained athletes and sportswomen, I do not recommend women to perform tummy exercises with weights. However, if you are really strong, there is no reason why you should not try Sit-ups (Exercise 14, Chapter 6) with a light disc held behind the head. I suggest a 2.3 kg (5 lb) disc to commence.

For actual training purposes you will need to select some of the exercises described above to make a well-balanced schedule. In the next chapter I have compiled a few simple exercise schemes to cater for most requirements. I hope you will try them.

Chapter 13

EXERCISE SCHEMES FOR ALL

By now you have received all the information needed to perform the exercises which will lead to new health and figure beauty.

Your problem is to decide which exercises to include in your training scheme. In this chapter I make some suggestions. Later on you will be able to construct your own schemes, but for a start I suggest you follow the advice given below.

I am going to assume that you start as a complete beginner, that you have no ailment which would make exercise unwise, and that you are neither very fat nor seriously underweight. I assume, also, that you have taken no serious exercise since you left school.

BEGINNERS' TRAINING SCHEME

Always start your exercise session with some warming-up freestanding work to loosen the muscles and prepare the system. These freestanding exercises are all described and illustrated in Chapter 6. The warm-up should last about five minutes and one set of each exercise should be sufficient. Try them in this order.

WARM-UP (FROM CHAPTER 6)
1. Stand astride, arms circling (Exercise 2).
2. Stand feet together, arms swing sideways and upwards (Exercise 3).
3. Stand astride, alternate toe touch (Exercise 6).
4. Leg forward raise (Exercise 11).

WEIGHT TRAINING (FROM CHAPTER 12)   Start with ten repetitions of each exercise. After about six training sessions try progressing to two sets of ten repetitions. Later go on to three sets of ten repetitions.
1. The Clean (Exercise 1).
2. Upright Rowing (Exercise 6).

3. The Squat (Exercise 19).
4. Straight Arm Pullover with Swingbell (Exercise 16).
5. Bench Press (Exercise 5).

TUMMY AND WAIST (FROM CHAPTER 6)   Always round
off your training scheme with tummy and waist exercises. But if
you think you may neglect this most important work, by all means
perform the exercises at an earlier stage. But they must be done –
every time without fail.
1. Neck rest, sidebends (Exercise 7).
2. Lie on back, alternate knee raise (Exercise 15).
3. Lying face downwards, neck rest, head and chest lift (Exercise
19).
4. Finish in the rest position for deep breathing (Exercise 21).

INTERMEDIATE TRAINING SCHEME

After you have performed the beginners' scheme correctly for some
twenty-five to thirty sessions you should be ready for something a
little more advanced.

You will notice that one or two exercises in the beginners'
scheme are still included. This is because certain exercises have
such great merit that they form a permanent part of nearly every
scheme, no matter how advanced. But you should now be able to
increase your weights on these old faithfuls, and also to attempt
three sets of ten repetitions.

WARM-UP (FROM CHAPTER 6)
1. Stand astride, arms forwards, arms swing sideways (Exercise 4).
2. Feet astride, alternate toe touch with both hands (Exercise 8).
3. Leg rest on chair or table, trunk forwards bend (Exercise 13).

WEIGHT TRAINING (FROM CHAPTER 12)
1. Press Behind Neck (Exercise 3).
2. The Squat (Exercise 19).
3. Straight Arm Pullover with Bar (Exercise 4).
4. Bench Press (Exercise 5).
5. Good Morning Exercise (Exercise 8).
6. Heels Raise, bar across front of thighs (Exercise 24).

TUMMY, WAIST AND BACK (FROM CHAPTER 6)
1. Lie on back, both knees raise to chest (Exercise 16).
2. Sit-ups (Exercise 14).
3. Resting weight on arms (front support), trunk lower (Exercise 9).
4. Finish in the rest position for deep breathing (Exercise 21).

ADVANCED TRAINING SCHEME

By the time you get to this stage you should be well aware of your own weak points. And you will be experienced enough to compile your own schemes to work on the areas that need concentrated attention.

Below, however, is an advanced general scheme. Loosen up as always, but the freestanding work should be limited so that you can attempt more weight training exercises.

WARM UP (FROM CHAPTER 6)
1. Feet astride, alternate toe touch with both hands (Exercise 8).
2. Quick Squats (Exercise 10).
3. Quick Sidebends (Exercise 7).

WEIGHT TRAINING (FROM CHAPTER 12)
1. Seated Press (Exercise 2).
2. Bent Over Rowing (Exercise 7).
3. Flying with Dumbells (Exercise 14).
4. Front Squat (Exercise 20).
5. Forward Lunge (Exercise 21).
6. Swingbell Swing (Exercise 18).

TUMMY, WAIST AND HIPS (FROM CHAPTER 6)
1. Front support, back lower (Exercise 9).
2. Lying on back, legs raise (Exercise 17).
3. Lying on back, high hip support, cycling (Exercise 18).
4. Finish in the rest position for deep breathing (Exercise 21).

FIFTEEN-MINUTE SCHEME

The three exercise schemes given may take between thirty and forty minutes to perform, depending on the number of repetitions attempted.

But suppose you are pressed for time one day, and can only spare fifteen to twenty minutes? There is no need to abandon any idea of training. It is surprising how much exercise you can get through in that short space of time. You will still be able to exercise every muscle group in the body.

That is the wonderful thing about weight training, of course. By playing games, or any other activity, it might take you two or three hours to get through the same amount of exercise. Here is a scheme that you can perform comfortably in fifteen to twenty minutes.

WARM UP (FROM CHAPTER 6)
1. Feet together, arms swing sideways and upwards ten times (Exercise 3).
2. Sidebends (Exercise 7).

WEIGHT TRAINING (FROM CHAPTER 12)   Perform one set of ten repetitions of each exercise.
1. Good Morning Exercise (Exercise 8).
2. The Squat (Exercise 19).
3. Bent Over Rowing (Exercise 7).

TUMMY AND WAIST (FROM CHAPTER 6)
1. Knees raise to chest (Exercise 16).
2. Sit ups (Exercise 14).

DUMBELL SCHEMES

It is possible that you may only possess dumbells. when travelling, for instance, they are less bulky than the long barbell rod. But you can still compile any number of varied and progressive schemes for this equipment. Here are two – one for beginners and one for the more advanced trainers.

BEGINNERS' DUMBELL SCHEME

WARM UP (FROM CHAPTER 6)
1. Feet astride, arms sideways, circling (Exercise 2).

2. Alternate toe touch (Exercise 6).
3. Leg swing sideways (Exercise 12).

DUMBELL TRAINING (FROM CHAPTER 12)
1. Alternate Dumbell Press, standing (Exercise 11).
2. The Squat (Exercise 26).
3. Straight Arm Pullover with swingbell (Exercise 16).
4. Forward Swing with swingbell (Exercise 18).
5. Lateral Raise sideways with discs (Exercise 17).

TUMMY, WAIST AND BACK (FROM CHAPTER 6)
1. Lying on back, alternate knee raise to chest (Exercise 15).
2. Toe touching from seated position (Exercise 14).
3. Prone lying head and chest raise (Exercise 19).
4. Finish in the rest position for deep breathing (Exercise 21).

ADVANCED DUMBELL SCHEME

WARM UP (FROM CHAPTER 6)
1. Stand, arms swing sideways (Exercise 4).
2. Feet astride, touch instep with both hands (Exercise 8).
3. Leg outstretched on chair or table, forwards bend (Exercise 13).

DUMBELL TRAINING (FROM CHAPTER 12)
1. Seated Alternate Dumbell Press (Exercise 12).
2. The Squat (Exercise 26).
3. Flying with dumbells (Exercise 14).
4. Sidebends with dumbells (Exercise 13).

TUMMY, WAIST AND HIPS (FROM CHAPTER 6)
1. Front support, body lower (Exercise 9).
2. Lying on the back, legs raise (Exercise 17).
3. Lying on back, high hip support, cycling (Exercise 18).
4. Finish in the rest position (Exercise 21).

SPECIALISATION

If you have poor thighs, bulky hips, or some other weak point, you will naturally want to devote more time to remedying these defects.

But you must still perform general exercises, adding extra work where you feel it is needed to build up or reduce.

Let us look at the weight training exercises described in Chapter 12 and note the ones which have the most effect on particular parts of the body.

BUST
1. Upright Rowing (Exercise 6).
2. Bent Over Rowing (Exercise 7).
3. Straight Arm Pullover (Exercise 4).
4. Bench Press (Exercise 5).
5. Flying with dumbells (Exercise 14).
6. Lateral Raise with discs (Exercise 17).
7. The Squat (Exercise 19). Remember, I said that this was a great stamina and chest builder, apart from its effect on the thighs.

LOWER BACK
1. Good Morning Exercise (Exercise 8).
2. Stiff-Legged Dead Lift (Exercise 9).
3. The Squat (Exercise 19). There is also a great deal of back work in this fine exercise.

THIGHS AND HIPS
1. Forward Lunge (Exercise 21).
2. Stiff-Legged Dead Lift (Exercise 9).
3. The Squat and Front Squat (Exercises 19 and 20).
4. Swingbell Swing (Exercise 18).
Plus all the iron-boot exercises.

SHOULDERS, ARMS, UPPER BACK
1. Seated Press (Exercise 2).
2. Press Behind Neck (Exercise 3).
3. Lateral Raise (Exercise 15).
4. Alternate Press with dumbells (Exercise 11).
5. Seated Alternate Press with dumbells (Exercise 12).
6. Straight Arm Pullover (Exercise 4).
The above exercises are excellent for posture, round shoulders, etc.

LOWER LEG
All the heels raise work (Exercises 23, 24, 25).

UPPER ARM

1. Curl (Exercise 10). Can also be performed seated with a swingbell, or with dumbells, etc.

Many of the upward pressing exercises, of course, have a marked effect on the arms.

TUMMY

The exercises I recommend for the tummy do not come under weight training. You will find them listed in Chapter 6.

1. Sit ups (Exercise 14).
2. Lying on the back, Alternate Knee Raise (Exercise 15).
3. Lying on the back, Both Knees Raise (Exercise 16).
4. Lying on the back, Both Legs Raise (Exercise 17).
5. Lying on the back, Cycling (Exercise 18).

Chapter 14

WEIGHT TRAINING FOR SPORT AND ATHLETICS

After the 1948 Olympic Games, held in London, the leading figures in British athletics decided to take a long, cool look at the training techniques practised by athletes in Britain.

Their reasons were not hard to find. Our own athletes possessed a high degree of skill, co-ordination and speed. But these qualities, alone, were no longer sufficient to win gold medals in world competition. Physical strength had become an essential factor, and there was every indication that American and European athletes had succeeded in building strength without in the process losing other necessary qualities.

At a now historic meeting, officials of the Amateur Athletic Association of Great Britain witnessed demonstrations of weight training exercises designed to assist athletes, and later, experiments were conducted with various athletes.

Now almost all athletes – men and women, whatever their event or sport – almost certainly use weight training or resistance exercises at some time during their training, especially in the off season. It is not only the shot putters, hammer throwers and weight lifters. Even great runners like Sebastian Coe and Allan Wells use quite heavy weight training exercises during their off season, and Daley Thompson certainly does.

Many top women athletes and sportswomen do also. Ann Jones, former Wimbledon Singles Champion, used resistance exercises for two seasons before she won her title, at a time when it had not become fashionable, and she was thinking of retiring from top tennis.

All physical education colleges include weight training in their syllabus. When I was at the army PT school at Aldershot, weight training was frowned upon, now they have weights and resistance machines, and it is all part of the training scheme for instructors.

At first, the top coaches tried to devise complicated routines for each event or sport, but it soon became evident that in general the basic exercises, properly applied, would suit almost any sport.

There was, of course, concentration on certain exercises which helped a weakness in a muscle group that needed building up or strengthening.

Many exercises are used for remedial purposes and for helping to build up muscle strength after injury. But we read that there is a dirth of physical medicine specialists among the British medical profession. Many top sports coaches tell us that this is where Britain is sadly lacking compared with other countries.

One or two big hospitals even had special athletes' clinics which were invaluable, and sportspeople with all sorts of injuries could get expert advice, but owing to cuts, many of these have had to close down. One does not expect the ordinary practitioner to be too conversant with the complex type of sports injuries, unless he has been a sportsman himself. A good osteopath is very valuable in this respect, but you must be sure he has experience and is properly qualified.

When training for athletics, or some particular sport, it is tempting to concentrate solely on the muscle groups most in need of strengthening for that event. But the other muscle groups must never be neglected, or the all-round strength so essential for success in modern sport will not be acquired, and there is always a danger of one-sided development.

I am convinced that many of the joint and muscle injuries suffered by women athletes are caused through lack of all-round training. Certain muscle groups are overworked, while the opposite groups are neglected and become weak and unable to stand sudden strain. Basic exercises for over-all strength and development will mould a more attractive figure, increase stamina and minimise the risk of muscular and joint injuries.

In this chapter I am going to suggest certain basic exercises to assist all sports, and also some individual exercises to aid particular events. Do not expect anything new. Many of the movements were standard weight training exercises known to me long before athletes discovered them. The athletes tend to forget that physical culturists have been using weight training methods for many years. But exercises are like fashions; they go in cycles of popularity and pop up over and over again. Only the terminology and methods of application change.

If you will refer back to Chapter 12 you will see that all the basic weight training exercises are fully described and illustrated, and they will not, therefore, be described again. I shall just give the name and number of each recommended exercise so that you can turn back to Chapter 12 yourself for full details.

As always, you must warm up before attempting weight training. Most athletes have their pet methods of limbering up, but there is a very good selection of suitable exercises in Chapter 6 for you to choose from. Spend at least five minutes on this work. The movements for tummy, waist and hips, along with the iron-boot exercises, will prove most beneficial.

Now for those basic exercises. Here they are, and I recommend them as first-class assistance movements for all sports and athletic events.

These exercises can be done in the form of circuit training, and many coaches recommend this form of training. Instead of doing, say, three sets or ten repetitions of each exercise, you work round a circuit of six to eight exercises doing one set of each, going round the circuit as fast as possible. You can time how long it takes to complete a circuit and chart your improvement. It is a good way of adding speed to strength, as long as the performance of each exercise does not suffer for the sake of improving your speed in their performance.

1. The Squat (Exercise 19) or Front Squat (Exercise 20).
2. Bench Press (Exercise 5).
3. Good Morning Exercise (Exercise 8).
4. Upright Rowing (Exercise 6).
5. Straight Arm Pullover (Exercise 4).
6. Any heels raise movement (Exercises 22, 23, 24 and 25).

These simple exercises are the basis of every training scheme for all sports and events. They will produce strength and stamina without reducing speed or co-ordination. They must be performed in strict style and through a full range of movement. I assume that as a sportswoman you are already fit, so you should not be afraid to handle reasonably heavy weights. If in doubt, start off with the figures suggested in Chapter 12 and see how you go.

Work on the set system, performing three sets of eight to ten repetitions of each exercise, and completing one exercise before starting the next. (For a full explanation of the set system see Chapter 11.) If you are an athlete and in training you will be able to perform higher repetitions on calf and tummy work.

As I have said, the exercises are described in full in Chapter 12, but let us examine each one and see why it is of particular importance to the athlete.

1. THE SQUAT (EXERCISE 19)   All athletes and sportswomen need strong legs. Many an athlete has been let down by pulled or strained thigh muscles, or by cramp. Power, even for throwing events, comes from the drive in the legs, plus the speed and co-ordination of the leg movements, whether in the run-up or in a circle. The thighs are served by some of the greatest and strongest muscle groups of the entire body.

The Squat is the best possible exercise for all the thigh muscles. It also boosts the respiratory system, so strengthening the heart and increasing lung power. It is a great chest builder and producer of stamina as well as a leg strengthener.

For all sports the Squat is a must. It builds power. For sprinters I suggest the Jumping Squat (Exercise 27), and higher and faster repetitions of the ordinary Squat.

2. BENCH PRESS (EXERCISE 5)   It is a fine chest and stamina builder and exercises the whole of the respiratory system. It also works the chest, arm and shoulder muscles. You can perform the Bench Press with fairly heavy weights without risk of injury as long as you follow the correct style.

It is particularly useful for the throwing events, for fencing, and for any sport in which a racket, stick or club is used. It is useful for swimming, too.

3. GOOD MORNING EXERCISE (EXERCISE 8)   This strengthens the lower back, a vulnerable trouble spot if at all weak. Because it stretches and strengthens the backs of the thighs and the 'hamstrings', the Good Morning Exercise is ideal for runners, jumpers and throwers and swimmers, but it is an all-round movement beneficial to everyone. (The Stiff-Legged Dead Lift, Exercise 9, can also be used if further back strength is required.)

4. UPRIGHT ROWING (EXERCISE 6)   This is a fine chest, forearm, shoulder and upper back exercise. Because it brings into play so many of the major muscle groups of the upper body. I consider it a most superior exercise when training for all sports and athletic events.

5. STRAIGHT ARM PULLOVER (EXERCISE 4)   Mobilises and strengthens the whole of the rib box and builds up the respiratory system. It also gives full range of movement to the shoulder girdle, and has a marked effect on the muscles at the backs of the arms and the large muscle groups of the upper body.

Instead of taking the bar to arms' length (as explained in the description) make a full movement by taking the bar or swingbell right to the thighs. This is a fine exercise for swimmers and throwers and anyone who needs added shoulder and back strength.

6. HEELS RAISE (EXERCISES 22, 23, 24, 25) I suggest a wide variety of exercises for the lower legs. For every sport they need all the strength they can get. Calves are very prone to injury, as are the Achilles tendons at the backs of the heels. Strengthen them to resist damage.

I suggest very high repetitions on these lower leg exercises – up to three sets of twenty – but do not perform more than two of the exercises in any one training session.

In the six basic exercises described above you have all you need to work a training scheme which will improve your performance in any form of sport. I know champion athletes who use only the Squat and the Straight Arm Pullover, and derive great benefit from even this limited form of work.

But let us, finally, consider a few other exercises which can be added to the basic list to assist in training for certain specialised events.

SPRINTING, THROWING EVENTS, BADMINTON, SQUASH, GOLF AND SWIMMING

Alternate Dumbell Press (Exercise 11) and Alternate Seated Dumbell Press (Exercise 12). They bring greater strength to shoulders, arms, forearms and wrists. They add power to the sprinter's arm movements, increase throwing power in field events, strengthen the swimmer's shoulders and arms. For golf and racket games they increase valuable forearm strength.

Lateral Raise with dumbells (Exercise 15). A very advanced shoulder exercise which also works the upper back. It is ideal for specialists in the events listed above.

JUMPING, FENCING AND FIELD EVENTS

Sidebends with dumbells (Exercise 13). For any event in which there is twisting and turning of the body, the lateral muscles must be strong. Sidebends will strengthen the whole of the vital area round the waist and lateral muscles.

Forward Lunge (Exercise 21). Ideal for fencers, this is particularly good for thighs and hip strength.

To round-out your scheme you may like to include the Curl (Exercise 10). It is an upper-arm strengthener of great value, and will compensate for exercises such as Straight Arm Pullover and Alternate Dumbell Press, in which the muscles at the backs of the arms are mostly used.

All the iron-boot exercises described in Chapter 11 are useful for the athlete; they strengthen the hips, tummy muscles and thighs.

Chapter 15

CORRECT BREATHING

Most garages have a notice up on the wall which reads 'Free Air'. Sometimes I think I would like to see the same sign exhibited in our great parks and open spaces.

Breath is life. Yet most people go through the day starved of air. They just do not know how to make full use of their lungs. Shallow breathing means that the extremities of the lungs never get any exercise. They become weak and open to infection and disease.

Pollution is a modern hazard, especially if you are a city dweller. This makes it all the more essential to try to breathe correctly as often as you can. Even the parks are better than busy streets, and the countryside or seaside are certainly a godsend to repair the damage done by daily breathing in of foul air and cigarette smoke.

Do always breathe correctly through your nose when not exercising, but through your mouth when doing strenuous exercise as you need a quicker intake of oxygen as you burn it up more quickly.

Try at all times, whatever you are doing, to breathe fully and deeply. The human body needs an adequate supply of oxygen more than anything else. You can live for several days without food and water, but you will not live for more than a few moments without air.

You will notice that I have laid great stress on correct breathing technique when describing exercises in this book. Please do follow my instructions implicitly on this point. You will never make much progress with your figure training if your breathing is faulty.

When you take exercise oxygen is burnt up very fast indeed. It is essential that you breathe deeply to maintain an adequate supply. If you should feel a little giddy or faint after the completion of an exercise don't be alarmed. You have not done yourself any harm. You are just suffering from temporary shortage of oxygen. A few deep breaths will put you right. That is one of the reasons why a short rest is recommended between exercises.

If you are really short of breath at the end of an exercise you will have to take in large gulps of air through the mouth, but normally it is much better to breathe in and out through the nose. This organ acts as a filter of dust and other impurities, and in cold weather it warms the air before it is taken into the lungs.

You will recall that at the end of every exercise I suggest you adopt a rest position – lying on the back, knees raised, feet flat on the floor, hands at sides with palms on floor. In this totally relaxed position you should breathe in and out slowly and deeply. Fill the lungs from bottom to top until you can breathe in no longer; then exhale equally slowly. When you think the lungs are really empty try to force just a little more air out of them.

Because the abdominal muscles are completely relaxed, this exercise is recommended for expectant mothers.

Many of the freestanding exercises described in Chapter 6 are particularly good as breathing exercises. Try these four.
1. Stand astride, arms circling (Exercise 2).
2. Stand feet together, arms raise sideways and up (Exercise 3).
3. Alternate toe touch, passing through the upright position (Exercise 8).
4. Lying on the back, pullover with a book (Exercise 5).

All these exercises can safely be performed after childbirth, and the first two are particularly recommended for expectant mothers. They will prove most beneficial. Even women of quite an advanced age can derive benefit from the first two exercises.

With all breathing exercises it is important to remember that exhalation is as important as inhalation. So breathe in fully; then exhale fully. Always make sure, too, that the nasal passages are clear. If deep breathing becomes a natural habit you will be a long way along the road to constant good health and freedom from colds. Exercise will help you make correct breathing a habit.

It is, after all, a basic instinct. When we come out of a stuffy building the first thing we do is to take a couple of deep breaths. We do the same when visiting the country or the sea. Try taking a few deep breaths on the way to the bus in the mornings, or after coming out of the office or cinema.

If you are out for a walk, try breathing in slowly and fully for ten paces, then out again for another ten. Do this for a short spell. You will be surprised how well it makes you feel.

Correct breathing alone will improve your posture and lift and mould the bust. It will brighten your complexion and give you a feeling of general well-being.

Chapter 16

THE AGE FACTOR AND SOME EXERCISES FOR EXPECTANT MOTHERS

Two questions are often asked me by women about to take exercise. How late in life can one start? And up to what age can one continue?

There is no doubt that the older you are the harder it is to get into good physical condition, and even if you have kept fit all your life there comes a time when you must gradually ease down the amount of exercise taken. But many people can and do continue light freestanding exercises well into their seventies. A lot of the exercises in Chapter 6 are perfectly safe for women of this age.

The top age at which you can start depends so much on your general health and condition that it is impossible to give a specific answer. If you are grossly overweight, diet should come first, coupled with very light freestanding exercises. Quite frankly, if you are physically capable of performing light work, then no matter how old you are, the exercise should do you good.

If you are in any doubt, consult your doctor. But do remember that he is not a physical educationist, and he will naturally tend to be cautious. Ask him outright if you can lift weights and you will probably get 'No' for an answer, unless he happens to be familiar with modern exercise methods.

Don't condemn your doctor if he seems to be vague on the subject of progressive resistance exercise. So many people expect their doctors to be physical education experts – which they are not – but they will always be happy to give you sound advice on keeping well.

It is possible that you were quite athletic in your younger days, but I am afraid you cannot suddenly decide to continue where you left off. The older you get, the stiffer you get, and the harder it is to make a come-back. If you have gained much weight, exercise will put added strain on the vital organs, and you will have to proceed very carefully.

I have known men and women of over fifty who have taken up weight training and obtained excellent results, but they have not been overweight and have been in good general condition. The later you start, the slower you will have to proceed, but results will always show in the end.

Be particularly patient if you are overweight. It is easier to accumulate fat than to melt it away. You cannot expect to lose a lot of weight in a few weeks. To do so could be dangerous.

FIGURE BEAUTY AFTER CHILDBIRTH

Even in these modern times too many women still believe that childbirth will see the end of their attractive figures. What nonsense. I can tell you from my own personal dealings with hundreds of contests that most of our best-known beauty queens and model girls are married women with families. At least two world-famous beauty queens have won major titles only a few weeks after the arrival of a baby.

Women who have taken care of their figures should look even more radiant and beautiful after childbirth. There is no excuse at all for letting yourself go.

If you are expecting a baby do try to attend your local pre-natal clinic. You will be shown exercises which will ensure you an easier confinement and will help to restore your figure after the birth as quickly as possible.

The deep-breathing exercises described in the previous chapter can, of course, be continued to within three or four weeks of the arrival of the baby.

After the birth of the baby, you will want to rest. Though in hospital they will have you doing ante-natal exercises within a day or so. When you get home the problems of coping with a new addition to the family will keep you occupied.

If there are no complications, and you are reasonably healthy, I suggest you practise the following freestanding exercises from Chapter 6, which you can commence about six weeks after your confinement.

1. Feet together, alternate toe touch (Exercise 6).
2. Feet together, neck rest, bending from side to side (Exercise 7).
3. Hands on hips, knees bend and stretch (Exercise 10).
4. Feet together, arms stretch sideways and upwards (Exercise 3).
5. Lying on the back, alternate knee raise (Exercise 15).
6. Standing, alternate leg raise to waist height (Exercise 11).

Ten weeks after confinement you should be able to manage a few harder freestanding exercises. I suggest the following.
1. Stand feet together, arms swing sideways and backwards (Exercise 4).
2. Stand feet astride, alternate toe touch with both hands (Exercise 8).
3. On the hands, trunk lower (Exercise 9).
4. Hands on hips, knees bend and stretch (Exercise 10).
5. Sit ups (Exercise 14).
6. Lying on the back, both knees raise (Exercise 16).

Light weight training exercises from Chapter 12 can safely be commenced about four months after the confinement. Couple them, at first, with some freestanding exercises. I suggest the following weight training movements as being most suitable at this stage. Perform one set only of each.
1. Bench Press (Exercise 5).
2. Upright Rowing (Exercise 6).
3. Good Morning Exercise (Exercise 8).
4. Straight Arm Pullover (Exercise 14).
5. Flying with dumbells (Exercise 14).

If you are in good health, training with chest expanders or beach ball can also commence four months after the confinement.

CONTRACEPTIVES

The contraceptive pill is used by millions of women, and some find that they put on weight round the hips and waist as a side-effect of the pill. You should always consult your doctor about any problems concerning the pill, and have regular check-ups, but if the doctor feels that the pill suits you in all other respects, you may wish to continue in its use. A programme of exercises can help to keep the fatty tissue under control and keep your figure slender and in trim.